Acute Management of Autism Spectrum Disorders

Editors

MATTHEW SIEGEL
BRYAN H. KING

CHILD AND ADOLESCENT PSYCHIATRIC CLINICS OF NORTH AMERICA

www.childpsych.theclinics.com

Consulting Editor
HARSH K. TRIVEDI

January 2014 • Volume 23 • Number 1

ELSEVIER

1600 John F. Kennedy Boulevard • Suite 1800 • Philadelphia, Pennsylvania, 19103-2899

http://www.theclinics.com

CHILD AND ADOLESCENT PSYCHIATRIC CLINICS OF NORTH AMERICA Volume 23, Number 1
January 2014 ISSN 1056–4993, ISBN-13: 978-0-323-26382-5

Editor: Joanne Husovski
Developmental Editor: Stephanie Carter

Child and Adolescent Psychiatric Clinics of North America (ISSN 1056-4993) is published quarterly by Elsevier Inc., 360 Park Avenue South, New York, NY 10010-1710. Months of issue are January, April, July, and October. Business and Editorial Offices: 1600 John F. Kennedy Boulevard, Suite 1800, Philadelphia, PA 19103-2899. Periodicals postage paid at New York, NY and additional mailing offices. Subscription prices are $310.00 per year (US individuals), $491.00 per year (US institutions), $155.00 per year (US students), $360.00 per year (Canadian individuals), $598.00 per year (Canadian institutions), $200.00 per year (Canadian students), $430.00 per year (international individuals), $598.00 per year (international institutions), and $200.00 per year (international students). International air speed delivery is included in all *Clinics* subscription prices. All prices are subject to change without notice. **POSTMASTER:** Send address changes to *Child and Adolescent Psychiatric Clinics of North America*, Elsevier Health Sciences Division, Subscription Customer Service, 3251 Riverport Lane, Maryland Heights, MO 63043. **Customer Service: 1-800-654-2452 (U.S. and Canada); 314-447-8871 (outside U.S. and Canada). Fax: 314-447-8029. E-mail: JournalsCustomer Service-usa@elsevier.com (for print support) or journalsonlinesupport-usa@elsevier.com (for online support).**

Reprints. For copies of 100 or more of articles in this publication, please contact the Commercial Reprints Department, Elsevier Inc., 360 Park Avenue South, New York, New York 10010-1710 Tel.: 212-633-3874; Fax: 212-633-3820, E-mail: reprints@elsevier.com.

Child and Adolescent Psychiatric Clinics of North America is covered in *MEDLINE/PubMed (Index Medicus), ISI, SSCI, Research Alert, Social Search, Current Contents,* and *EMBASE/Excerpta Medica.*

Printed and bound by CPI Group (UK) Ltd, Croydon, CR0 4YY

Transferred to digital print 2012

Contributors

CONSULTING EDITOR

HARSH K. TRIVEDI, MD
Associate Professor of Psychiatry, Vanderbilt University School of Medicine; Executive Medical Director, Chief of Staff, Vanderbilt Psychiatric Hospital, Nashville, Tennessee

CONSULTING EDITOR EMERITUS

ANDRÉS MARTIN, MD, MPH

FOUNDING CONSULTING EDITOR

MELVIN LEWIS, MBBS, FRCPSYCH, DCH

EDITORS

MATTHEW SIEGEL, MD
Director, Developmental Disorders Program, Spring Harbor Hospital, Maine; Assistant Professor of Psychiatry, Tufts University School of Medicine, Boston, Massachusetts; Clinical Investigator, Maine Medical Center Research Institute, Westbrook, Maine

BRYAN H. KING, MD
Director, Department of Psychiatry and Behavioral Medicine, Seattle Children's Autism Center, Seattle Children's Hospital; Professor and Vice Chair, Department of Psychiatry and Behavioral Sciences, University of Washington, Seattle, Washington

AUTHORS

MICHAEL G. AMAN, PhD
Ohio State University, Ohio

L. EUGENE ARNOLD, MD, MEd
Ohio State University, Ohio

KAREN BEARSS, PhD
Emory University, Georgia

CAROL BERESFORD, MD
Medical Director, Neuropsychiatric Special Care, Department of Psychiatry, University of Colorado Denver; Children's Hospital Colorado, Aurora, Colorado

THOMAS P. CAMPBELL, MD, MPH
Associate Professor, Temple University Medical School, System Chairman Emergency Medicine, West Penn Allegheny Health System, Pittsburgh, Pennsylvania

DEVON CARROLL, MSN
Family and Children's Aid, Danbury, Connecticut

NINA DE LACY, MD
Department of Psychiatry and Behavioral Sciences, University of Washington, Seattle, Washington

PETER DOEHRING, PhD
Director, ASD Roadmap, Chadds Ford, Pennsylvania

ROBIN L. GABRIELS, PsyD
Associate Professor, Department of Psychiatry, University of Colorado Denver; Program Director, Neuropsychiatric Special Care, Children's Hospital Colorado, Aurora, Colorado

JAN S. GREENBERG, PhD
Professor and Director, School of Social Work, Waisman Center Investigator, University of Wisconsin-Madison, Madison, Wisconsin

LOUIS HAGOPIAN, PhD
Director, Neurobehavioral Inpatient Unit, Department of Psychiatry and Behavioral Sciences, Johns Hopkins University School of Medicine, Baltimore, Maryland

VICTORIA HALLETT, PhD
Kings College in London, London, United Kingdom

BENJAMIN L. HANDEN, PhD, BCBA-D
Associate Professor of Psychiatry and Pediatrics, Western Psychiatric Institute and Clinic of UPMC, University of Pittsburgh School of Medicine; Associate Professor of Psychology and Education, Department of Psychology in Education, University of Pittsburgh, Pittsburgh, Pennsylvania

TODD HARRIS, PhD
Director of Autism Services, Devereux Pennsylvania, Downingtown, Pennsylvania

TIFFANY L. HUTCHINS, PhD
Assistant Professor, Department of Communication Sciences and Disorders, University of Vermont, Burlington, Vermont

CYNTHIA JOHNSON, PhD
University of Pittsburgh, Pittsburgh, Pennsylvania

BRYAN H. KING, MD
Director, Department of Psychiatry and Behavioral Medicine, Seattle Children's Autism Center, Seattle Children's Hospital; Professor and Vice Chair, Department of Psychiatry and Behavioral Sciences, University of Washington, Seattle, Washington

LUC LECAVALIER, PhD
Ohio State University, Ohio

MARTIN J. LUBETSKY, MD
Professor of Psychiatry, Clinical Service Chief, Child and Adolescent Psychiatry and Center for Autism and Developmental Disorders, Western Psychiatric Institute and Clinic of UPMC, Children's Hospital of Pittsburgh of UPMC, University of Pittsburgh School of Medicine, Pittsburgh, Pennsylvania

MICHELLE LUBETSKY, MEd, BCBA
Allegheny Intermediate Unit, Homestead, Pennsylvania

MARSHA R. MAILICK, PhD
Vaughan Bascom and Elizabeth M. Boggs Professor, Director, Waisman Center, University of Wisconsin-Madison, Madison, Wisconsin

CARLA A. MAZEFSKY, PhD
Assistant Professor, Department of Psychiatry, University of Pittsburgh School of Medicine, Pittsburgh, Pennsylvania

JAMES T. MCCRACKEN, MD
University of California at Los Angeles, Los Angeles, California

CHRISTOPHER J. MCDOUGLE, MD
Harvard University, Massachusetts

JOHN J. MCGONIGLE, PhD
Assistant Professor of Psychiatry, Western Psychiatric Institute and Clinic of UPMC, University of Pittsburgh School of Medicine; Assistant Professor of Rehabilitation Science Technology, University of Pittsburgh School of Health and Rehabilitation Sciences, Pittsburgh, Pennsylvania

CAROL ANNE MCNELLIS, PsyD
Clinical Director, Devereux Pennsylvania Children's ID/D Services, West Chester, Pennsylvania

TAMARA PALKA, MD
Attending Psychiatrist, Developmental Disorders Unit, Foundations Behavioral Health, Doylestown, Pennsylvania

CARA PHILLIPS, PhD, BCBA
Postdoctoral Fellow, Neurobehavioral Inpatient Unit, Kennedy Krieger Institute, The Johns Hopkins School of Medicine, Baltimore, Maryland

PATRICIA A. PRELOCK, PhD, CCC-SLP
Professor, Department of Communication Sciences and Disorders, Dean, College of Nursing and Health Sciences, University of Vermont; Professor, Pediatrics, College of Medicine, University of Vermont, Burlington, Vermont

BRIAN REICHOW, PhD, BCBA-D
Associate Research Scientist, Child Study Center, Yale School of Medicine, New Haven, Connecticut

LAWRENCE SCAHILL, MSN, PhD
Emory University, Georgia

MATTHEW SIEGEL, MD
Director, Developmental Disorders Program, Spring Harbor Hospital, Maine; Assistant Professor of Psychiatry, Tufts University School of Medicine, Boston, Massachusetts; Clinical Investigator, Maine Medical Center Research Institute, Westbrook, Maine

LEANN E. SMITH, PhD
Assistant Clinical Professor of Pediatrics, Waisman Center Investigator, University of Wisconsin-Madison, Madison, Wisconsin

KIMBERLY A. STIGLER, MD
Department of Psychiatry, Christian Sarkine Autism Treatment Center, Riley Hospital for Children, Indiana University School of Medicine, Indianapolis, Indiana

DENIS G. SUKHODOLSKY, PhD
Yale University, Connecticut

NAOMI SWIEZY, PhD
Indiana University, Indiana

ELAINE TIERNEY, MD
Kennedy-Krieger in Baltimore, Baltimore, Maryland

ARVIND VENKAT, MD
Vice Chair for Research and Faculty Academic Affairs, Department of Emergency Medicine, West Penn Allegheny Health System, Pittsburgh, Pennsylvania

BENEDETTO VITIELLO, MD
National Institute of Mental Health, Maryland

SUSAN W. WHITE, PhD
Associate Professor, Department of Psychology, Virginia Tech, Blacksburg, Virginia

Contents

Children with autism spectrum and related disorders and intellectual disability are not protected from the experience of psychiatric illnesses. Many factors can contribute to exacerbation of existing behavioral symptoms or to the emergence of new psychiatric problems. The psychiatric assessment must thus take into account a range of possible etiologic or contributory factors. The approach outlined in this article highlights the value of assessing 4 broad domains, including diagnostic (genetic) factors, medical considerations, developmental influences, and environmental factors. Examples of how the consideration of each of these domains may inform the diagnostic formulation are highlighted.

The purpose of this article is to describe emotion regulation, and how emotion regulation may be compromised in patients with autism spectrum disorder (ASD). This information may be useful for clinicians working with children with ASD who exhibit behavioral problems. Suggestions for practice are provided.

Severe problem behaviors such as aggression, self-injury, and property destruction can result in injury, and require specialized and expensive treatment. This article reviews outcome research published since 1995 that used behavioral techniques to decrease severe problem behaviors among children and adolescents with autism spectrum disorder and/or intellectual disability. Many relatively simple interventions were reported to significantly reduce severe problem behavior, which offers hope for practitioners. Nonetheless, these studies also reveal a risk for injury and a need for specialized assessment and placement, careful tracking, and high-quality treatment that few agencies could likely replicate without increases in training and support.

This article describes the relationship between expressive communication
impairments and common challenging behaviors in individuals with Autism
Spectrum Disorder and Intellectual Disability. The communication challenges of individuals with Autism Spectrum Disorder/Intellectual Disability
are described and several evidence-based intervention strategies are proposed to support communication so as to decrease challenging behaviors.
Recommendations for practice are offered.

This study identified subtypes of aggression in a sample of 206 children
with autism spectrum disorder (ASD) who participated in 2 risperidone
trials. The narratives were derived from a parent interview about each
child's 2 most pressing problems. Five subtypes of aggression emerged:
hot aggression only, cold aggression only, self-injurious behavior (SIB)
only, aggression and SIB, and nonaggressive. All groups showed a high
rate of positive response to risperidone with no differences across subtypes. These study findings extend understanding of aggression in ASD
and may be useful to guide further study on biological mechanisms and
individualized treatment in ASD.

Individuals diagnosed with autism spectrum disorders (ASD) often exhibit
serious behavioral disturbance (irritability) including severe tantrums,
aggression, and self-injury that requires pharmacologic management.
Research focused on the treatment of severe irritability has primarily
involved the atypical antipsychotics, including risperidone and aripiprazole. Anticonvulsants have also been investigated for targeting serious
behavioral disturbance; however findings have been mixed. Advances in
the pharmacotherapy of irritability in ASD continue to inform practice.
Research is needed to develop safer and more effective drug treatments
for serious behavioral disturbance in this population.

Individuals with autism spectrum disorder (ASD) presenting with acute
agitation in emergency departments (ED) during a crisis situation present
both diagnostic and treatment challenges for ED personnel, families,
caregivers, and patients seeking treatment. This article describes the

challenges that individuals with ASD face when receiving treatment in crisis and emergency settings. Additionally, this article provides information
for emergency physicians, ED personnel, and crisis response teams on
a systematic, minimally restrictive approach when assessing and providing treatment to patients with ASD presenting with acute agitation in ED
settings.

Individuals with Autism Spectrum Disorder present with unique characteristics, and the interventions designed to address associated challenging
behaviors must be highly individualized to best meet their needs and those
of their families. This article reviews systems of care to support the child,
adolescent, or adult with Autism Spectrum Disorder and/or Intellectual
Disability. The review describes mental health/behavioral health services,
Intellectual Disability and other support systems, and the systems involved
in a child and adolescent's life and transition to adulthood. The types of
systems and services, as well as barriers, are delineated with a brief listing
of Web sites and references.

For children diagnosed with an autism spectrum disorder and/or intellectual disability, the co-occurrence of serious behavioral disturbance can
pose significant health and safety risks, impede normal learning and
development, and put great stress on family systems. The complexity
and seriousness of the clinical concerns often tax the existing service
and funding systems. Although residential treatment has been criticized
as an outdated and ineffective mode of treatment, newer models of
residential treatment that combine specialized comprehensive services,
evidence-based interventions, intensive family support and training, and
treatment overlap with community providers can offer an effective and
efficient treatment option.

Children with autism spectrum disorder are psychiatrically hospitalized
much more frequently than children in the general population. Hospitalization occurs primarily because of externalizing behaviors and is associated
with behavioral disturbance, impaired emotion regulation, and psychiatric
comorbidity. Additionally, a lack of practitioner and/or administrator training and experience with this population poses risks for denial of care by
third-party payers or treatment facilities, inadequate treatment, extended
lengths of stay, and poor outcomes. Evidence and best practices for the
inpatient psychiatric care of this population are presented. Specialized

treatment programs universally rely on multidisciplinary approaches, including behaviorally informed interventions.

Leann E. Smith, Jan S. Greenberg, and Marsha R. Mailick

This article reports the findings from a longitudinal program of research examining the bidirectional influences of the family environment on the behavioral phenotype of autism, and describes a newly developed family psychoeducation program, titled *Transitioning Together*, designed to reduce family stress, address behavior problems, and improve the overall quality of life of adolescents with autism and their families. A case study is presented that illustrates how *Transitioning Together* helps reduce family stress and improve the overall quality of the family environment. The article concludes with a discussion of directions for future research on best practices in working with families of children, adolescents, and adults with autism.

CHILD AND ADOLESCENT PSYCHIATRIC CLINICS

RELATED INTEREST

Brain, Behavior, and Immunity, March 2011 (Vol. 25, No. 3)
Autoantibodies to Cerebellum in Children with Autism Associate with Behavior
Paula Goines, Lori Haapanen, Robert Boyce, Paul Duncanson,
Daniel Braunschweig, Lora Delwiche, Robin Hansen, Irva Hertz-Picciotto,
Paul Ashwood, Judy Van de Water

AACAP Members: Please go to www.jaacap.org for information on access to the Child and Adolescent Psychiatric Clinics. *Resident* Members of AACAP: Special access information is available at www.childpsych.theclinics.com.

NOW AVAILABLE FOR YOUR iPhone and iPad

Preface

Autism and Developmental Disorders: Management of Serious Behavioral Disturbance

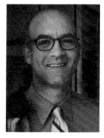 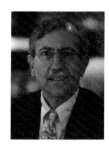

Matthew Siegel, MD   Bryan H. King, MD
Editors

This issue of the *Child and Adolescent Clinics of North America* tackles the area of serious behavioral disturbance in children and adolescents with Autism Spectrum Disorder (ASD) and Intellectual Disability (ID). Children who struggle with challenging behaviors, including aggression and self-injury, present some of the most significant clinical challenges for professionals in this field.

The authors of the articles that follow have captured the complexity of assisting these children and their families, while offering clear, practical approaches to improve outcomes. This issue of the *Child and Adolescent Clinics of North America* spans the major modalities for helping children with developmental disorders: from approaches utilizing psychopharmacology, communication supports, emotion regulation, family intervention, and behaviorism to treatment settings and systems, including outpatient, emergency room, residential, and inpatient care. It is our hope that the reader comes away from this text with a broad array of tools with which to approach and support children and families struggling with serious behavioral disturbance.

Psychiatric assessment of children and adolescents with ASD or ID is a complex endeavor, demanding the translation of traditional evaluation techniques into developmentally informed approaches. Drs King, de Lacy, and Siegel open the issue by outlining the best practices for psychiatric assessment of the population, including the evidence for use of standardized measures.

Child Adolesc Psychiatric Clin N Am 23 (2014) xiii–xv
http://dx.doi.org/10.1016/j.chc.2013.08.007
1056-4993/14/$ – see front matter © 2014 Elsevier Inc. All rights reserved.

childpsych.theclinics.com

Examining deficits in emotion regulation offers a broad, trans-diagnostic approach to challenges faced by the population. Drs Mazefsky and White provide an excellent review of the unique difficulties with emotion regulation experienced by children with ASD and encourage a focus on developing regulatory strategies that will reduce problem behaviors.

Applied behavioral treatments have some of the strongest evidence for efficacy in children with ASD and ID but have faced challenges in dissemination due to methodological issues related to the use of single subject trials. Drs Doehring, Reichow, Palka, Phillips, and Hagopian provide a fresh analysis of the behavioral literature that highlights efficacious approaches, identifying a focus on proactive behavioral techniques based on functional behavioral assessment.

Practitioners who work closely with the population recognize the primacy of communication, and in the words of our expert authors, "there is no distinction between communication and behavior." Drs Hutchins and Prelock efficiently articulate the barriers to communication experienced by those across the autism spectrum and review the evidence for communication interventions to reduce behavioral disturbance.

Although there is currently no psychopharmacologic treatment for the core symptoms of ASD, prudent use of medications can play an important role in addressing serious behavioral challenges. Dr Stigler masterfully captures the evidence for medication treatment and provides guidance for prescribing practices. In a related vein, Devon Carroll, MSN and Drs Hallet, Mcdougle, Scahill, and colleagues provide a new analysis of data from the seminal risperidone trials for children with autism and serious behavioral disturbance. They offer valuable new insights into potential subtypes of aggression and self-injury in ASD that may spur refinements in pharmacologic approaches.

Designing systems to help individuals with developmental disorders achieve their greatest potential in the least restrictive environment is the focus of increasing efforts on the federal, state, and local levels. Drs McGonigle, Venkat, Beresford, Campbell, and Gabriels offer insightful approaches for safely reducing acute behavioral disturbance in the emergency room and other settings. Drs Lubetsky, Handen, McGonigle and Michelle Lubetsky, MEd, BCBA then follow with a thoughtful analysis of the multiple systems of care needed to support individuals with developmental disorders and highlight a leading model developed with the State of Pennsylvania.

Psychiatric hospitalization of children with ASD or ID represents the most intensive of interventions but is frequently required in response to serious behavioral disturbance. Drs Siegel and Gabriels provide a comprehensive review of the evidence for treatment in general and specialized inpatient child psychiatry units and offer practical suggestions for adapting inpatient environments and approaches to the needs of the population.

Finally, Drs Smith, Greenberg, and Mailick illustrate the impacts of serious behavioral disturbance on families, and the role families may play in maintaining or ameliorating challenges. Following a line of longitudinal research spanning over 13 years, the authors offer their latest evidence for family intervention in ASD.

We wish to thank Joanne Husovski of Elsevier and consulting editor, Harsh Trivedi, MD, for their assistance in assembling this issue of the *Child and Adolescent Clinics of North America*. We would also like to thank Emily Siegel, PsyD, Girard Robinson, MD, and Donald L. St. Germain, M.D. (M.S.) and Ludwik Szymanski, MD, James Harris, MD, and Peter Tanguay, MD (B.K.) for their steadfast guidance and support of our work. We are uniquely blessed to be able to do the work we do with a special population.

Matthew Siegel, MD
Developmental Disorders Program
Spring Harbor Hospital
123 Andover Road
Westbrook, ME 04092, USA

Bryan H. King, MD
Department of Psychiatry and Behavioral Medicine
Seattle Children's Hospital
4800 Sand Point Way NE
Seattle, WA 98105, USA

E-mail addresses:
siegem@springharbor.org (M. Siegel)
bhking@u.washington.edu (B.H. King)

Psychiatric Assessment of Severe Presentations in Autism Spectrum Disorders and Intellectual Disability

Bryan H. King, MD[a,b,*], Nina de Lacy, MD[b],
Matthew Siegel, MD[c,d,e]

KEYWORDS

- Autism • Intellectual disability • Self-injury • Aggression • Hyperactivity
- Psychiatric evaluation

KEY POINTS

- Psychiatric illnesses are common in autism spectrum disorder (ASD)/intellectual disability (ID).
- Externalizing behaviors are common presenting symptoms but are etiologically nonspecific.
- Genetic conditions associated with ASD/ID may inform medical surveillance as well as potential therapeutics.
- Co-occurring medical conditions are common in ASD/ID and may contribute to symptom presentation.
- Environmental factors, for example, change in caregiver or experience of trauma, may be particularly significant in the setting of ASD/ID.

INTRODUCTION

Decades ago, Sovner and Hurley[1] somewhat rhetorically debated whether individuals with ID experience affective illness. Although the answer then as now is an unequivocal yes, uncertainty does remain as to how the presentation of psychiatric

Disclosure Statement: B.H. King has received research funding and has served as a consultant for Seaside Therapeutics and Roche. Drs N. de Lacy and M. Siegel report no financial disclosures.

[a] Department of Psychiatry and Behavioral Medicine, Seattle Children's Autism Center, Seattle Children's Hospital, Seattle, WA, USA; [b] Department of Psychiatry and Behavioral Sciences, University of Washington, Seattle, WA, USA; [c] Developmental Disorders Program, Spring Harbor Hospital, ME, USA; [d] Tufts University School of Medicine, Boston, MA, USA; [e] Maine Medical Center Research Institute, ME, USA
* Corresponding author.
E-mail address: bhking@u.washington.edu

Child Adolesc Psychiatric Clin N Am 23 (2014) 1–14
http://dx.doi.org/10.1016/j.chc.2013.07.001
1056-4993/14/$ – see front matter © 2014 Elsevier Inc. All rights reserved.

childpsych.theclinics.com

disorders may be altered in the setting of atypical intellectual development. More-over, as the genetic underpinnings of neuropsychiatric illness are revealed and certain behavioral phenotypes elaborated in association with particular genetic abnormalities, questions have been raised about the appropriateness of applying nonspecific illness labels to behaviors that occur in specific contexts. In cases of hyperphagia and restricted interests in Prader-Willi syndrome, for example, is value added by superimposing the psychiatric diagnoses of impulse control disorder or obsessive-compulsive disorder?

Conversely, there is every bit as much heterogeneity in symptom expression in the context of genetic syndromes as for the general population. Not everyone with Prader-Willi syndrome has significant skin-picking behavior nor does Lesch-Nyhan syndrome guarantee aggression, although these are common symptom-syndrome correlations. Taking a step back, the same can be said for persons with idiopathic ID: not everyone with severe ID is aggressive, self-injurious, or hyperactive. These problems occur only in a minority of this population.

Howe[2] observed that "there are some among the lowest class of idiots who seem to have a superabundance of innervation, who are consequently very active. They appear like insane persons in a state of excitement, and yet they have no speech, and no reasoning faculties."[2] Hurd,[3] who was superintendent of the Eastern Michigan Asylum, wrote that irritability, violence, and impulsivity alone are insufficient grounds for the diagnosis of insanity in this "lowest grade of imbeciles," but impulsive acts, "morbid propensities," and "acts of suicidal intent" (eg, "attempting to dash one's brains"), "occurring in higher grades of imbecility" are symptoms consistent with "actual insanity," even in the absence of delusions.

The recognition that even severe ID neither protects nor precludes an individual from experiencing psychiatric illness is thus one of the earliest observations from clinicians working in this field. Modern studies generally estimate that having ID increases the risk of psychiatric illness at least 3-fold or 4-fold relative to the general population,[4,5] thereby underscoring the importance of careful psychiatric assessment in this population.

PREVALENCE OF PSYCHIATRIC ILLNESS

Estimates of the overall prevalence of psychiatric disorders in individuals with ID range from 10% to 39%.[6,7] In children and adolescents, emotional and behavioral problems occur up to 7 times more frequently than in typically developing youth.[8]

Specific factors that place individuals with ID at increased risk for developing comorbid psychopathology include severity of disability, lower adaptive behavior, language impairments, poor socialization, low socioeconomic status, and families with only 1 biologic parent.[9] In general, developmental and genetic disorders are associated with elevated rates of depression and anxiety. Specific genetic syndromes are also associated with increased rates of particular disorders, such as higher rates of depression in Down syndrome (DS),[10] anxiety, and ADHD in individuals with Williams syndrome and increased rates of schizophrenia in velocardiofacial syndrome (22q11.2 deletion syndrome).[11,12]

Psychiatric illness is also clearly more prevalent in the ASD population than in the general population. Prevalence estimates vary based on the type of measure used. When diagnostic instruments developed for the neurotypical population are used for individuals with ASD, high rates of comorbid psychiatric illness are found. Using the Kiddie Schedule for Affective Disorders and Schizophrenia (K-SADS) for School-Age Children,[13] in a psychiatrically referred population, produced an estimate of

6.4 comorbid psychiatric diagnoses in each child with ASD.[14] Similarly, using the Structured Clinical Interview for DSM-IVTR (SCID)[15] in adults with ASD resulted in diagnosing 60% to 70% of subjects with depression and anxiety.[16] Instruments adapted for the ASD population produce lower estimates, such as rates of anxiety and depression of 10% to 44% in children with ASD.[17]

REASONS FOR REFERRAL FOR PSYCHIATRIC ASSESSMENT

Although psychiatric illnesses are common in the setting of ID, it is the presence of severe behavioral problems that typically prompt referral for psychiatric evaluation. King and colleagues[18] analyzed the chief complaints from 251 consecutive psychiatric referrals in an institutionalized population with mostly severe to profound ID. Behavioral disturbances accounted for upwards of 80% of reasons for referral, with the remainder representing a collection of medical concerns (eg, rule out tardive dyskinesia and assess current medication regimen). As can be seen in **Fig. 1**, self-injurious behavior, aggression, hyperactivity, and impulsivity top the list.

N = 251 Consecutive Psychiatric Consultations in an Institutional Setting

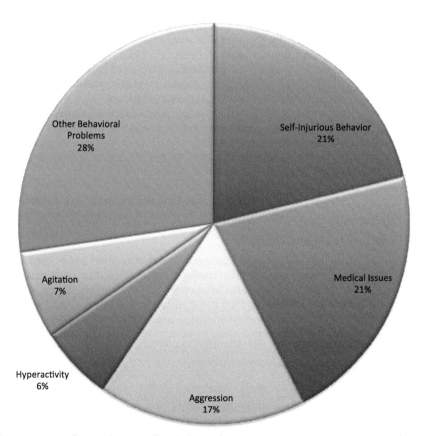

Fig. 1. Reasons for psychiatric referral. (*Data from* King BH, De Antonio C, McCracken JT, et al. Psychiatric consultation in severe and profound mental retardation. Am J Psychiatry 1994;151(12):1802–8.)

More recently, Siegel and colleagues[19] examined the reasons for psychiatric admission to a specialized inpatient service for children and adolescents with autism and related conditions. In this population requiring acute stabilization for severe behavioral disturbance, aggression and self-injurious behavior predominated.

These severe behavioral presentations are heterogeneous from the standpoint of their diagnostic etiology, and comorbidity among them is common. The approach to the assessment for each of these behavior targets is not exclusive but must clearly be comprehensive. Siegel and Gabriels highlight the variety of potential contributing factors to symptom presentation in the setting of ASD/ID. (See the article by Siegel and Gabriels elsewhere in this issue for further exploration of this topic.)

GENERAL ASSESSMENT ISSUES

Assessment of psychiatric disorders in children and adolescents typically involves several variables, including a child's own description of symptoms and experiences; descriptions from parents, teachers, or other care providers; and direct observations of behavior.

Language Skills and Communication Development

Because of often limited language development and communication skills and symptom presentation that may differ from that observed in the absence of intellectual impairments, interviews with family, teachers, and other caregivers regarding their observations and assessment of nonverbal aspects of behavior take on a more critical role in evaluating mental disorders in this population. It is also of particular importance to clinicians to construct a picture of a child's baseline level of cognitive and executive functioning, emotional expressivity, and language development. With respect to the latter, it is important to distinguish between receptive and expressive language skills, because these may be different. It is not unheard of, for example, to be astounded that a minimally verbal youngster takes a ride on the Internet like a professional, navigating text menus and entering search terms with ease. Many parents are appropriately sensitive to the possibility that discussing all of the problems that brought a child in to the hospital or clinic within earshot of the child may, at a minimum, be uncomfortable for many patients—and, on occasion, agitate the child and prompt or elicit behavioral disturbances like those being discussed.

Accommodations Made by Caregivers

Interviews of children with ASD/ID and their caregivers may need to be adapted to capture relevant information. Similar to cases of obsessive-compulsive disorder, family systems frequently accommodate behaviors and symptoms of a child in order to minimize disruption and maintain homeostasis within the family unit. It is, thus, sometimes necessary to identify and subtract out accommodation to gain an appreciation for the true level of dysfunction. Questions, such as "What would happen if you insisted John get off the computer?" and "How would John react if you did bring him into the store?" may provide a more full picture.

Clinician Questions

Questions asked in an interview of a patient should be short, simple, and to the point and asked one at a time with ample time allotted for processing of the information. Whenever possible, the clinician should attempt to verify the comprehension of the question in order to avoid successive "yes" or "no" answers. Similarly, echolalic responses can be checked by switching the order of the variables: "Are you happy or sad?" and then "Are you sad or happy?" Clinicians should be aware that some individuals with developmental delay might seek to please and thus answer in the affirmative if they do not understand the question or know the answer.[20] In addition, clinicians should avoid leading questions. For example, if a child with ID is asked whether he/she hears voices, most positive responses refer to normal internal self-talk. Instead children could be asked if they hear things others people in the room do not hear. In particular, self-report questionnaires have been found frequently unreliable in the ID population due to problems with question content, question phrasing, and response format.[21]

Comorbidities

Comorbid medical and neurologic conditions are also germane to psychiatrists, in particular, the presence of epilepsy, metabolic/mitochondrial disorders, and autoimmune, gastrointestinal, and endocrine illness.

A comprehensive assessment thus encompasses several potential etiologic dimensions, including

Diagnostic
Medical
Developmental
Environmental

In the following sections, these dimensions are reviewed, including case vignettes focusing on some of the most common presenting behavioral symptoms to child psychiatrists.

DIAGNOSTIC CONSIDERATIONS

As discussed previously, knowledge of the underlying cause of an ID or ASD may be helpful in informing the psychiatric work-up and ongoing management. ASD and ID are increasingly understood as common or shared neurobehavioral outcomes of hundreds of underlying genetic conditions[22] disrupting molecular pathways involved in organogenesis and organ function, including, but not necessarily limited to, the brain. ASD and ID may be associated with single gene variants or copy number variants that might have an impact on any 1 of dozens of relevant genes with an array of neurobehavioral and somatic consequences. These genetic events can have complex neuropsychiatric implications. For example, a clinician caring for DS patient wants to place early-onset Alzheimer dementia on the differential for an individual with disruptive behavior and likewise check thyroid, visual, and hearing function in the presence of mood disturbance, because DS carries well-established risks for such problems.[23] More subtle effects are also potentially important in this population. For example, patients with genetic syndromes have higher rates of perinatal birth complications and those with congenital cardiac or other defects may undergo multiple early surgeries, incurring the concomitant neurobehavioral risks of repeated anesthesia.[24]

More recently, as genes are identified and the pathophysiology associated with genetic disruption is elaborated and understood, potential targets for intervention and rational pharmacologic treatment are also revealed. Genetic and molecular diagnosis ultimately assist in parsing diagnostic options with more specificity.

As a case in point, fragile X syndrome (FXS) and tuberous sclerosis complex (TSC) are both disorders that significantly increase the risk for ASDs. FXS is a trinucleotide repeat disease affecting the *FMR1* gene, which, in its full expression, may account for approximately 5% of ASD cases[25] and is the most common heritable cause of ID.[26] Symptoms of autism appear in 20% to 50% of individuals with FXS.[27,28] ADHD symptoms and executive function deficits are also common,[29,30] and the developmental trajectory of attention and working memory more broadly is significantly delayed compared with typically developing individuals.[31] Increasingly, it is understood that premutation carriers under 200 repeats may also manifest with ASD and other psychiatric disorders.[22] The gene defect in FXS is associated with an excitatory/inhibitory imbalance in the synapse,[32] likely resulting from upregulation of glutamatergic spine formation and a concomitant hyperexcitable state.

The gene defect in TSC affecting hamartin or tuberin also results in an excitatory inhibitory imbalance, and up to 60% of patients have ASD.[33–35] The imbalance is in the opposite direction, however, likely resulting from activation of the PI3K/mTOR pathway. The disorders associated with TSC are similar to those in FXS, including ADHD, aggression, and epilepsy,[36,37] neatly illustrating how similar neurobehavioral outcomes can be produced by opposed microstructural mechanisms. Mouse models seem to confirm this opposition.[38]

Although still preliminary, these findings suggest the presence of a Goldilocks phenomenon in which the balance of excitation and inhibition needs to be "just right." The imbalances created in certain genetic syndromes, which may present with similar behavioral symptoms, may actually require different, even opposite approaches, as when the problem is "too cold" or "too hot." Emerging, specific treatments for ASD in the context of FXS may actually exacerbate ASD symptoms in disorders like TSC and vice versa.

Thus, newer research is targeting the specific pathways involved in TSC and FXS,[39–41] offering the prospect of more rationally defined therapies and underlining the importance of accurate diagnosis at the genetic-molecular level. More broadly, a similar phenomenon is found in other monogenic conditions and polygenic copy number variants, where loss or gain of function mutations and deletions or duplications can produce similar phenotypes. Increasingly, therefore, the identification of the genetic condition underlying ID or ASD informs treatment selection given behavioral phenotype alone cannot discriminate molecular mechanism.

In patients with an identified genetic diagnosis, consultation of the literature can be helpful to psychiatrists in suggesting treatment. Many genetic syndromes have a neuropsychiatric signature, although phenotypic severity and presentation also often vary widely for reasons that are incompletely understood. Furthermore, it is common to see the neurobehavioral presentation in neurogenetic disorders evolve over time, sometimes changing radically over the neurodevelopmental arc through early adulthood. Clinicians want to continue reassessment, adjusting behavioral interventions, medications, and dosages accordingly.

In patients without a diagnosis, genetic assessment is a first-line recommendation[42] in both ASD and ID. In the authors' institution, the Comparative Genomic Array Hybridization (CGH) + Single Nucleotide Polymorphisms (SNP) array is the most common first line general assay. FXS testing is often added for ID and ASD. Where there is high suspicion based on phenotype for a particular disorder, Fluorescence In Situ Hybridization testing may be substituted where available given its ease and affordability.

MEDICAL CONSIDERATIONS

The importance of considering potential medical contributions to the expression of severe behavioral disturbance cannot be overstated where behavioral change is often the canary in the coal mine of an underlying medical condition. Studies have repeatedly demonstrated that co-occurring medical conditions are common, perhaps even to be expected, as a result of the condition that underlies the neurodevelopmental disorder. For example, Charlot and colleagues[43] observed that 60% of individuals with ID admitted to their specialized inpatient service for severe behavior disorders had constipation, and 38% had gastroesophageal reflux. With respect to risks associated with particular syndromes, the craniofacial abnormalities and immune system deficits forming part of the common phenotype of 22q.11 deletion/velocardiofacial syndrome (the most common survivable genetic deletion syndrome) frequently lead to recurrent otitis media.[44]

In cases of idiopathic ID and ASD, medical problems as commonplace in childhood as constipation, tooth pain, or ear infection can initially present as severe behavioral exacerbations.[45] Furthermore, chronic comorbidities, such as autoimmune, endocrinologic, cardiac, or gastrointestinal disorders, are common in those with genetic syndromes. The specific genetic deficit underlying an ASD or ID may involve basic physiologic pathways involved in homeostasis, basic metabolism, stress response, and immune and inflammatory mechanisms: many mechanisms could account for behavioral exacerbations during illness or stress flares. For example, the deleterious neuropsychiatric effects of physiologic stress on children with mitochondrial or metabolic disorders (associated with ID and ASD in some cases)[46] are well known in clinical practice and may require buffering with sick day management. Clinicians should also be alert to the possibility for anticipating medication or dosage adjustment during puberty, growth spurts, or weight changes.

Many individuals with moderate to severe ID and ASD are nonverbal or have highly impaired expressive language and may have extreme baseline sensory sensitivity or insensitivity. Thus, clinicians are presented with both the challenges of engaging such individuals in regular physical examinations (eg, it can be challenging to look in the ear of someone with extreme sensory sensitivity) and the fact that many individuals have limited or no ability to tell care providers that they are in pain or to help localize the site of their discomfort. Thus, psychiatrists must be vigilant for possible medical problems presenting as behavioral problems in this population. Opportunities should be sought to package assessments (eg, during required anesthesia or conscious sedation) and maintain excellent preventative medical care hand in hand with psychiatric care optimization. It is encouraging to see that several initiatives are under way to support general health maintenance for the population with ID.[47,48]

Another important factor to consider is the potential behavioral toxicity of medications used to treat co-occurring conditions. Many individuals with ASD and related conditions also have epilepsy for example, and the potential adverse impact of an anticonvulsant in terms of increasing irritability, adversely affecting mood, or diminishing impulse control and contributing to behavioral activation is well established.[49] Children with comorbid conditions requiring the use of medications for pulmonary, cardiac, or gastroenterologic symptoms, such as calcium channel blockers, phosphodiesterase inhibitors, and centrally acting antiemetics or muscle relaxants, are also at high risk of neurobehavioral side effects.

In this context, virtually any psychotropic drug can contribute to behavioral disturbance in some individuals, and it is important to consider possible alternative medical strategies as potentially more helpful than parallel and competing approaches with psychiatric drugs. Close coordination with providers, particularly the prescribing neurologist, is clearly of benefit.

CASE VIGNETTE: AGITATION/IMPULSIVITY

Presentation: A 12-year-old girl with Smith-Lemli-Opitz syndrome is brought in for an emergent appointment by her parents because she is becoming increasingly dysregulated and agitated, including attempts to dart away from her parents in public places. She has low expressive verbal ability and cannot explain what is wrong but does appear agitated and labile.

Work-up

Diagnostic: molecular testing previously performed

Medical: Complete blood count + differential, electrolytes, urinalysis, lipid panel

Developmental: long history of developmental delay and ASD but no recent changes

Environmental: no changes in caregivers, history of abuse, or other recent disruption

Results: urinalysis shows greater than 100,000 colony-forming units of Escherichia coli and many white cells; complete blood count shows white blood cell count of 19.

Management: in consultation with her primary care physician and the biochemical genetics department, as her primary inpatient psychiatrist you decide to pursue hospital admission. After several days of antibiotics, a steroid burst and optimization of her cholesterol dietary supplements her agitation is much improved. Psychiatric medications are left unchanged, but note is made to avoid haldoperidol because it exacerbates cholesterol abnormalities in Smith-Lemli-Opitz syndrome.[50]

DEVELOPMENTAL CONSIDERATIONS

Human development is a path-dependent process with every future state affected by past state. From conception onwards, genome and environment interact in a continuous bidirectional process mediated by the brain. Individuated patterns of genetic expression progressively unfold over the long human neurodevelopmental arc into young adulthood, reflecting unique combinations of genomic variation (and mutation) with environmental experience. Over time, these patterns specify the sequential construction and growth of brain structures from which behaviors emerge, also in temporally patterned sequences recognizable as characteristic developmental periods and milestones. Long-term synaptic potentiation and the creation of brain internetworks serve to stabilize mature skills and memories and inhibit juvenile or unneeded behaviors.

Cognition (defined here as learning and memory) and behavioral development are, therefore, inextricably intertwined throughout development. Individuals' general intellectual ability modifies their ability to learn, remember, and reproduce new behaviors and knowledge. Furthermore, humans learn most importantly through social learning; thus, those individuals with impaired social cognition as occurs in ASD experience problems in acquiring new behaviors associated with these deficits. There is well-validated support for the notions that ID is associated with or increases risk for neurodevelopmental disorders, including ASD, attention-deficit/hyperactivity disorder (ADHD), and schizophrenia[51] and, conversely, that higher general cognitive function is a predictor of better psychiatric outcomes in these disorders. Petersen and colleagues[52] have shown that language ability, independent of other measures of cognitive function, uniquely contributes to the risk for behavior problems in children.

Thus, there are perhaps 2 major dimensions that might be encompassed under developmental dimensions of assessment. One is to consider where a given patient is on a developmental continuum, that is, what is reasonable to expect in terms of learning and behavior. Do individuals' IDs place them on a different trajectory, where what might be a concerning symptom in a typically developing child—for example, the persistence of rigidity or hitting into the kindergarten years—merely reflects a slower timetable? A second, related question to ask is to what degree is the problem behavior or symptom expression a reflection of what has been learned?

Psychiatric diagnoses may, therefore, be somewhat malleable in light of what is expected for developmental level given the degree of ID. This is the essential idea of developmental delay as distinct from ID. It is the same principle that underlies the qualifiers in *Diagnostic and Statistical Manual of Mental Disorders* criteria for certain disorders (eg, that the symptoms being manifest are in excess of, or atypical, in light of the individuals developmental age).

ADHD is a paradigmatic example of a neurobehavioral disorder that must be viewed in a developmental context. It is the most commonly diagnosed neuropsychiatric disorder among persons with ID.[53,54] Cardinal symptoms of course include inattention, impulsivity, and hyperactivity with onset before age 12, reflecting the expectation that in a typically developing child these behaviors are increasingly suppressed during the early school years as the prefrontal cortex matures, supporting the development of stronger executive function. ADHD has its own developmental course in typically developing children, with hyperactivity dominating earlier and inattention more prominent in the preteen years.[55] Lower cognitive function appears likely to exacerbate and lengthen symptoms and there is evidence that the presence of ID increases the risk for ADHD.[56]

Perhaps similar to Sovner and Hurley's rhetorical running of affective disorders up the flagpole in ID, historically, it has occasionally been considered superfluous to diagnose ADHD in the presence of ID. Over the years, some investigators[57–59] have argued that ADHD symptoms in this population are merely outgrowths of restricted cognition. Recent studies by Neece and colleagues,[53,56] however, compared ADHD in children and adolescents with ID and typical development and found that ADHD was a clinically and functionally valid diagnosis as a distinct comorbidity of ID. Individuals with ID experienced a similar developmental course with respect to symptoms of hyperactivity but, unlike typically developing children, who exhibited an increase and then decrease in inattentive symptoms in the teen years, persons with ID had no change in these symptoms, supporting the idea that lower cognitive function is at least correlated with persistent inattentive ADHD.

ENVIRONMENTAL CONSIDERATIONS

Changes to environment or social setting can be important triggers to acute behavioral crisis and decompensation in persons with ASD and ID. Individuals with ASD and ID may be particularly sensitive to changes in their environments, given common issues, such as behavioral rigidity, stereotyped interests and routines, difficulty with transitions, sensory sensitivity, and impulsivity. Acute decompensation may be precipitated by a change in routine or setting, loss of a caregiver or friend, or even dietary or housing changes. Lower levels of general cognitive function can make adaptation to change and learning challenging or more prolonged. In a study that explored precipitating events associated with crisis visits to an emergency department, Lunsky and Elserafi[60] found 6 stressful life events that were significant predictors of a likely emergency visit. These events were move of house or residence; a serious problem with family, friend or caregiver; problems with police or other authorities; sustained unemployment; recent trauma/abuse; and drug or alcohol problem. Other studies have shown that the risk for trauma in ID is elevated throughout the lifespan.[61]

Inasmuch as ID is a risk factor for psychiatric illness, the importance of environmental factors on trajectory and outcome cannot be overstated. Many studies have examined various contributors to quality of life in persons with ID. Factors like independence, self-determination, interpersonal relation,s and social inclusion all importantly influence quality of life.[62]

A robust literature highlights the importance of environmental factors on the development and maintenance of behaviors that can be maladaptive.[63] Hitting or biting may be an effective way to gain or keep something of importance, and these behaviors play out in preschools all over the world. As these and related behaviors are reinforced in the environment, they may become particularly problematic over time. Systematic and detailed assessment of the potential functions that behaviors serve is a critical part of the assessment of these symptoms in the setting of ASD/ID. Behavioral analysis and related interventions are highlighted elsewhere in this issue by Doehring and colleagues.

CASE VIGNETTE: AGGRESSION

Presentation: a 17 year-old nonverbal adolescent with autism is brought in by his mother and older sister (who happened to be visiting from out of state) for evaluation of aggressive behavior. He has been hospitalized on 3 occasions for attempting to stab the care providers in his group home. During each hospitalization he is described as calm; there is virtually no aggression evident in the hospital setting.

Work-up

Diagnostic: molecular testing previously performed and noncontributory

Medical: recent routine laboratory testing was normal but a weight gain of 20 lb was noted at last outpatient visit attributed to a change in appetite associated with receipt of olanzapine initiated during previous hospital stay.

Developmental: patient seems to have better receptive than expressive language and was diagnosed with ASD early in life. He has a history of significant aggressive and self-injurious behavior, which eventually prompted his out-of-home placement.

Environmental: he has been relatively stable until approximately 2 years ago, however, when his group home changed.

A detailed history of the events that had resulted in hospitalization, all of which seemed to happen entirely out of the blue and when the patient seemed to be in particularly good spirits, prompted his sister to remember a childhood game she and her brother played in the home. The game, monsters, involved one of the kids taking a table knife from the kitchen and chasing the other through the house until caught and then everyone falling down and switching roles. This information resulted in a significant reconceptualization of the knife wielding behavior that had resulted in emergency hospitalizations and a successful behavioral intervention strategy.

SUMMARY AND FUTURE DIRECTIONS IN ASD/ID

Children with ASD/ID present myriad challenges to diagnosticians with respect to the complexity of psychiatric presentation and the seemingly innumerable potential factors that might contribute to symptom expression. Furthermore, the unraveling of these issues is often complicated by communication impairments, developmental variation, and co-occurring medical problems.

This article approaches this complexity by focusing on 4 broad dimensions that inform the approach to evaluation and treatment in ASD/ID. Through the consideration of known genetic factors, medical conditions, developmental influences, and environmental factors, clinicians will be well positioned to move forward with the ongoing assessment and treatment of these challenging conditions.

REFERENCES

1. Sovner R, Hurley AD. Do the mentally retarded suffer from affective illness? Arch Gen Psychiatry 1983;40(1):61–7.
2. Howe SG. Report made to the legislature of Massachusetts upon Idiocy. Boston: Coolidge and Wiley; 1848. p. 64.
3. Hurd HM. Imbecility with insanity. Am J Insanity 1888;45:261–9.
4. Dekker MC, Koot HM, van der Ende J, et al. Emotional and behavioral problems in children and adolescents with and without intellectual disability. J Child Psychol Psychiatry 2002;43(8):1087–98.
5. Emerson E, Einfeld S. Emotional and behavioural difficulties in young children with and without developmental delay: a bi-national perspective. J Child Psychol Psychiatry 2010;51(5):583–93.
6. Borthwick-Duffy SA. Epidemiology and prevalence of psychopathology in people with mental retardation. J Consult Clin Psychol 1994;62(1):17–27.
7. Bouras N, Drummond C. Behaviour and psychiatric disorders of people with mental handicaps living in the community. J Intellect Disabil Res 1992;36(Pt 4): 349–57.
8. Dykens EM. Psychopathology in children with intellectual disability. J Child Psychol Psychiatry 2000;41(4):407–17.
9. Koskentausta T, Iivanainen M, Almqvist F. Psychiatric disorders in children with intellectual disability. Nord J Psychiatry 2002;56(2):126–31.
10. Collacott RA, Cooper SA, McGrother C. Differential rates of psychiatric disorders in adults with Down's syndrome compared with other mentally handicapped adults. Br J Psychiatry 1992;161:671–4.
11. Gothelf D, Frisch A, Michaelovsky E, et al. Velo-cardio-facial syndrome. J Ment Health Res Intellect Disabil 2009;2(2):149–67.
12. Green T, Avda S, Dotan I, et al. Phenotypic psychiatric characterization of children with Williams syndrome and response of those with ADHD to methylphenidate treatment. Am J Med Genet B Neuropsychiatr Genet 2012;159B(1):13–20.
13. Kaufman J, Birmaher B, Brent D, et al. Schedule for affective disorders and schizophrenia for school-age children – present and lifetime version (K-SADS-PL): initial reliability and validity data. J Am Acad Child Adolesc Psychiatry 1997;36(7): 980–8.
14. Joshi G, Petty C, Wozniak J, et al. The heavy burden of psychiatric co-morbidity in youth with autism spectrum disorders: a large comparative study of a psychiatrically referred population. J Autism Dev Disord 2010;40:1361–70.
15. First MB, Spitzer RL, Williams JB, et al. Structured clinical interview for DSM-IV-TR (SCID-I) – research version. New York: Biometrics Research, New York State Psychiatric Institute; 2002.
16. Joshi G, Wozniak J, Petty C, et al. Psychiatric comorbidity and functioning in a clinically referred population of adults with autism spectrum disorders: a comparative study. J Autism Dev Disord 2013;43(6):1314–25.
17. Leyfer OT, Folstein SE, Bacalman S, et al. Comorbid psychiatric disorders in children with autism: interview development and rates of disorders. J Autism Dev Disord 2006;36:849–61.
18. King BH, DeAntonio C, McCracken JT, et al. Psychiatric consultation in severe and profound mental retardation. Am J Psychiatry 1994;151(12):1802–8.
19. Siegel M, Doyle K, Chemelski B, et al. Specialized inpatient psychiatry units for children with autism and developmental disorders: a United States survey. J Autism Dev Disord 2012;42(9):1863–9.

20. Sigelman CK, Budd EC, Spanhel CL, et al. When in doubt say yes: acquiescence in interviews with mentally retarded persons. Ment Retard 1981;19:53–8.

21. Finlay WM, Lyons E. Methodological issues in interviewing and using self-report questionnaires with people with mental retardation. Psychol Assess 2001;13: 319–35.

22. de Lacy N, King BH. Revisiting the relationship between autism and schizophrenia: toward an integrated neurobiology. Annu Rev Clin Psychol 2013;9: 555–87.

23. Glasson EJ, Dye DE, Bittles AH. The triple challenges associated with age-related comorbidities in Down syndrome. J Intellect Disabil Res 2013. [Epub ahead of print]. http://dx.doi.org/10.1111/jir.12026.

24. Flick RP, Katusic SK, Colligan RC, et al. Cognitive and behavioral outcomes after early exposure to anesthesia and surgery. Pediatrics 2011;128(5):e1053–61.

25. Budimirovic DB, Kaufmann WE. What can we learn about autism from studying fragile X syndrome? Dev Neurosci 2011;33(5):379–94.

26. Saul RA, Tarleton JC. FMR1-Related Disorders. 1998 Jun 16 [Updated 2012 Apr 26]. In: Pagon RA, Adam MP, Bird TD, et al, editors. GeneReviews™ [Internet]. Seattle (WA): University of Washington, Seattle; 1993–2013. Available at: http://www.ncbi.nlm.nih.gov/books/NBK1384/.

27. Hatton DD, Sideris J, Skinner M, et al. Autistic behavior in children with fragile X syndrome: prevalence, stability, and the impact of FMRP. Am J Med Genet A 2006;140A(17):1804–13.

28. Gabis LV, Baruch YK, Jokel A, et al. Psychiatric and autistic comorbidity in fragile X syndrome across ages. J Child Neurol 2011;26(8):940–8.

29. Sullivan K, Hatton D, Hammer J, et al. ADHD symptoms in children with FXS. Am J Med Genet A 2006;140(21):2275–88.

30. Van der Molen MJ, Van der Molen MW, Ridderinkhof KR, et al. Attentional set-shifting in fragile X syndrome. Brain Cogn 2012;78(3):206–17.

31. Cornish K, Cole V, Longhi E, et al. Mapping developmental trajectories of attention and working memory in fragile X syndrome: developmental freeze or developmental change? Dev Psychopathol 2013;25(2):365–76.

32. Gatto CL, Broadie K. Genetic controls balancing excitatory and inhibitory synaptogenesis in neurodevelopmental disorder models. Front Synaptic Neurosci 2010;2:4.

33. Wiznitzer M. Autism and tuberous sclerosis. J Child Neurol 2004;19(9):675–9.

34. Wong V. Study of the relationship between tuberous sclerosis complex and autistic disorder. J Child Neurol 2006;21(3):199–204.

35. Numis AL, Major P, Montenegro MA, et al. Identification of risk factors for autism spectrum disorders in tuberous sclerosis complex. Neurology 2011;76(11):981–7.

36. Chung TK, Lynch ER, Fiser CJ, et al. Psychiatric comorbidity and treatment response in patients with tuberous sclerosis complex. Ann Clin Psychiatry 2011;23(4):263–9.

37. Muzykewicz DA, Newberry P, Danforth N, et al. Psychiatric comorbid conditions in a clinic population of 241 patients with tuberous sclerosis complex. Epilepsy Behav 2007;11(4):506–13.

38. Auerbach BD, Osterweil EK, Bear MF. Mutations causing syndromic autism define an axis of synaptic pathophysiology. Nature 2011;480(7375):63–8.

39. Sahin M. Targeted treatment trials for tuberous sclerosis and autism: no longer a dream. Curr Opin Neurobiol 2012;22(5):895–901.

40. Kohrman MH. Emerging treatments in the management of tuberous sclerosis complex. Pediatr Neurol 2012;46(5):267–75.

41. Wijetunge LS, Chattarji S, Wyllie DJ, et al. Fragile X syndrome: from targets to treatments. Neuropharmacology 2013;68:83–96.
42. Schaefer GB, Mendelsohn NJ. Clinical genetics evaluation in identifying the etiology of autism spectrum disorders: 2013 guideline revisions. Genet Med 2013;15(5):399–407.
43. Charlot L, Abend S, Ravin P, et al. Non-psychiatric health problems among psychiatric inpatients with intellectual disabilities. J Intellect Disabil Res 2011;55(2): 199–209.
44. Ford LC, Sulprizio SL, Rasgon BM. Otolaryngological manifestations of velocardiofacial syndrome: a retrospective review of 35 patients. Laryngoscope 2000; 110(3 Pt 1):362–7.
45. Woods R. Behavioural concerns–assessment and management of people with intellectual disability. Aust Fam Physician 2011;40(4):198–200.
46. Dhillon S, Hellings JA, Butler MG. Genetics and mitochondrial abnormalities in autism spectrum disorders: a review. Curr Genomics 2011;12(5):322–32.
47. Lennox N, Bain C, Rey-Conde T, et al. Effects of a comprehensive health assessment programme for Australian adults with intellectual disability: a cluster randomized trial. Int J Epidemiol 2007;36(1):139–46.
48. Gordon LG, Holden L, Ware RS, et al. Comprehensive health assessments for adults with intellectual disability living in the community - weighing up the costs and benefits. Aust Fam Physician 2012;41(12):969–72.
49. Kerr M, Gil-Nagel A, Glynn M, et al. Treatment of behavioral problems in intellectually disabled adult patients with epilepsy. Epilepsia 2013;54(Suppl 1):34–40.
50. Nowaczyk MJM. Smith-Lemli-Opitz Syndrome. 1998 Nov 13 [Updated 2013 Jun 20]. In: Pagon RA, Adam MP, Bird TD, et al, editors. GeneReviews™ [Internet]. Seattle (WA): University of Washington, Seattle; 1993–2013. Available at: http://www.ncbi.nlm.nih.gov/books/NBK1143/.
51. Cristino AS, Williams SM, Hawi Z, et al. Neurodevelopmental and neuropsychiatric disorders represent an interconnected molecular system. Mol Psychiatry 2013. [Epub ahead of print]. http://dx.doi.org/10.1038/mp.2013.16.
52. Petersen IT, Bates JE, D'Onofrio BM, et al. Language ability predicts the development of behavior problems in children. J Abnorm Psychol 2013;122(2): 542–57.
53. Neece CL, Baker BL, Blacher J, et al. Attention-deficit/hyperactivity disorder among children with and without intellectual disability: an examination across time. J Intellect Disabil Res 2011;55(7):623–35.
54. Baker BL, Neece CL, Fenning RM, et al. Mental disorders in five-year-old children with or without developmental delay: focus on ADHD. J Clin Child Adolesc Psychol 2010;39(4):492–505.
55. Willoughby MT. Developmental course of ADHD symptomatology during the transition from childhood to adolescence: a review with recommendations. J Child Psychol Psychiatry 2003;44(1):88–106.
56. Neece CL, Baker BL, Crnic K, et al. Examining the validity of ADHD as a diagnosis for adolescents with intellectual disabilities: clinical presentation. J Abnorm Child Psychol 2013;41(4):597–612.
57. Gjaerum B, Bjornerem H. Psychosocial impairment is significant in young referred children with and without psychiatric diagnoses and cognitive delays–applicability and reliability of diagnoses in face of co-morbidity. Eur Child Adolesc Psychiatry 2003;12(5):239–48.
58. Reiss S, Valenti-Hein D. Development of a psychopathology rating scale for children with mental retardation. J Consult Clin Psychol 1994;62(1):28–33.

59. Tonge BJ, Einfeld SL, Krupinski J, et al. The use of factor analysis for ascertaining patterns of psychopathology in children with intellectual disability. J Intellect Disabil Res 1996;40(3):198–207.
60. Lunsky Y, Elserafi J. Life events and emergency department visits in response to crisis in individuals with intellectual disabilities. J Intellect Disabil Res 2011; 55(7):714–8.
61. Martorell A, Tsakanikos E, Pereda A, et al. Mental health in adults with mild and moderate intellectual disabilities: the role of recent life events and traumatic experiences across the life span. J Nerv Ment Dis 2009;197(3):182–6.
62. Claes C, Van Hove G, Vandevelde S, et al. The influence of supports strategies, environmental factors, and client characteristics on quality of life-related personal outcomes. Res Dev Disabil 2012;33(1):96–103.
63. Matson JL, Kozlowski AM, Worley JA, et al. What is the evidence for environmental causes of challenging behaviors in persons with intellectual disabilities and autism spectrum disorders? Res Dev Disabil 2011;32(2):693–8.

Emotion Regulation
Concepts & Practice in Autism Spectrum Disorder

Carla A. Mazefsky, PhD[a],*, Susan W. White, PhD[b]

KEYWORDS

- Emotion regulation • Autism spectrum disorder • Therapy • Behavioral problems
- Review

KEY POINTS

- Emotion regulation (ER) involves modulating the temporal features, intensity, or valence of one's emotions in the service of adaptive or goal-directed behavior.
- Disrupted ER may be inherent in autism spectrum disorder (ASD).
- Impaired ER may be a more parsimonious explanation than psychiatric comorbidity for severe behavioral disturbances observed in ASD.
- Few interventions have been developed to explicitly target ER processes in ASD.
- ER may be addressed (even if not labeled as such) in some existing psychosocial treatments used in ASD, including the provision of positive behavioral supports, enhancing emotional language, and modified cognitive–behavioral therapy.
- Areas of future need include the development and validation of measures to assess ER in ASD for treatment planning and evaluation purposes, as well as the development of interventions to promote ER that incorporate the unique characteristics of ASD.

INTRODUCTION
Emotion Regulation Concepts

Imagine that you are driving to work, and someone cuts you off. Your heart rate rapidly increases, and you experience a wave of intense irritation, yet you manage to blare on your horn, simultaneously hit your brakes, and remain focused on safely driving. You have just engaged in effective emotion regulation (ER), which broadly encompasses the processes related to modifying one' emotions to fit the context or meet one's goals[1,2] (in this case, staying safe). Although the distinction is widely debated,[3–5] emotion regulation differs from the experience of emotion itself, in that ER involves an attempt to modify the intensity or temporal features of an emotion (eg, after the

Funding: NICHD K23CHD060601 (C.A. Mazefsky); NIMH K01MH079945 (S.W. White).
Conflicts of Interest: None.
[a] Department of Psychiatry, University of Pittsburgh School of Medicine, University of Pittsburgh, 3811 O'Hara Street, Webster Hall, Suite 300, Pittsburgh, PA 15213, USA; [b] Department of Psychology, Virginia Tech, 109 Williams Hall (0436), Blacksburg, VA 24061-0100, USA
* Corresponding author.
E-mail address: mazefskyca@upmc.edu

Child Adolesc Psychiatric Clin N Am 23 (2014) 15–24
http://dx.doi.org/10.1016/j.chc.2013.07.002
1056-4993/14/$ – see front matter © 2014 Elsevier Inc. All rights reserved.

initial startle when you are cut off, you quickly experience anger when you see the driver texting [emotion], but, you attempt to keep the anger from escalating so that you can remain focused on safely driving [ER]). ER processes can occur at the unconscious level (without realizing you are doing so, you maintain a level of fear that will keep you alert but not unable to act) and at a conscious level (eg, telling yourself you are okay after the incident is over). Further, ER can be response-focused as in this example, or antecedent-focused (prior to the emotion).

Most people have a characteristic and fairly stable ER style. A person's customary ER style can be generally adaptive or maladaptive, with the latter often associated with psychopathology and less appropriate behavior. Disrupted, or maladaptive, ER has been implicated as a mechanism underlying various psychiatric disorders, including depressive[6,7] and anxiety[8] disorders and borderline personality disorder.[9] Thus, poor ER is a transdiagnostic process that plays a role in many disorders in producing inappropriate emotional and behavioral reactions. The mechanisms that give rise to emotional dysregulation and how ER manifests itself, however, are more disorder-specific.[9]

Role of ER in Autism Spectrum Disorder

Although much less studied in autism spectrum disorder (ASD) than in other psychiatric disorders, disrupted ER is likely to be a significant factor in producing aberrant behavior in ASD as well.[10,11] One likely manifestation of ER failure in ASD is serious behavioral disturbance. Tantrums, uncontrolled outbursts, aggression, and self-injury are often interpreted as defiant or deliberate. Although this interpretation is likely accurate in some circumstances, it is more often the case that these inappropriate behavioral reactions stem from ineffective management of emotional states in response to stress or overstimulation.[12]

Absent or impaired ER may be a more parsimonious explanation of serious behavioral disturbance in ASD than psychiatric comorbidity. Psychiatric diagnoses are difficult to reliably make in ASD for a variety of reasons, including lack of measures validated for use with this population, difficulty assessing certain symptoms in nonverbal individuals, inadequate insight and poor temporal reporting, unique manifestations of distress in ASD, and the challenges involved in interpreting and differentiating symptoms that could be attributed to ASD or a secondary disorder (eg, lack of positive affect as part of ASD or because of depression).[13,14] For all of these reasons, there is growing concern that psychiatric diagnoses may be overused in ASD.[15] Many secondary psychiatric problems may be more accurately conceptualized as part of the ASD itself or may stem from a fundamental problem in ER.[10]

ASD-Related Factors that Impede Effective ER

Many characteristics of ASD may interfere with effective ER (**Fig. 1**).[16] First, alexithymia, or difficulty identifying, distinguishing, and describing emotions, has been well documented in ASD.[17–19] Although not essential for all forms of ER, recognizing and understanding one's own emotions is necessary for effortful ER.[20] Labeling of one's emotion has been proposed as critical to successful ER,[21] and being able to communicate to others about one's emotional state is also involved in interpersonal ER aspects, such as joint problem solving or sharing of one's emotions. Given that language competence is associated with emotional competence in typical development,[22] it is also conceivable that the language and communication impairments common in ASD affect development or regulatory abilities.

As proposed by Samson, Huber, and Gross,[23] core deficits in theory of mind, or ability to take others' perspectives cognitively and effectively and to recognize one's own state of mind, may be related to poor ER. Some regulatory strategies

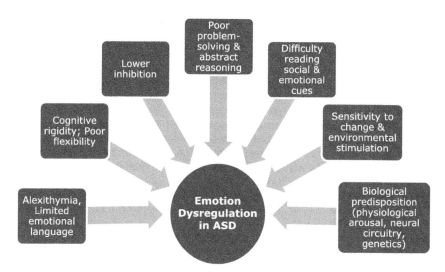

Fig. 1. Characteristics of ASD that may contribute to emotion dysregulation.

(eg, intentionally changing one's cognitive frame or perspective) are inherently related to perspective-taking ability. The social and cognitive deficits that define ASD also create ER challenges, particularly given that adaptive ER is context-dependent and requires one to be able to accurately identify critical aspects of the situation.[10] Even among cognitively higher-functioning individuals with ASD, there are deficits in the processing and integration of complex information.[24] Children with ASD may focus on the wrong information or misinterpret others' intentions because of failures in perspective taking and lack of appreciation of others' perceptions and experiences (eg, theory of mind deficits),[25] which could increase frustration. Difficulty accurately perceiving others' social and emotional cues may also interfere with the timing and implementation of effortful ER strategies. Impulsivity and impaired inhibition, which are present in as many as 50% of children with ASD,[26] could similarly interfere with ER. Specifically, even if the child knows what he or she should do when upset (eg, take deep breaths), inability to inhibit the more potent and automatic response (eg, hitting and yelling) could result in ineffective ER. If a child with ASD does stop to think about the situation before reacting, the tendency to be rigid and engage black-and-white thinking may still preclude a flexible and adaptive ER response.[10] Even on structured neuropsychological tests in laboratory settings (which are slower and more straightforward than the fast-moving interactions that require ER in daily life), problem-solving deficits in ASD have been documented.[24]

Finally, children with ASD may be predisposed to problems with emotional control given differences in arousal and underlying neural circuitry. Children with ASD are known to have unusual reactions to sensory information and are often sensitive to change. These differences in responses to the environment may increase reactivity and lability.[27] Further, although results are not entirely consistent, there is evidence to suggest that at least some of the ASD population is physiologically hyperaroused,[28] particularly those who present with anxiety symptoms. Additionally, although neuroimaging research on ER in ASD is limited, there is evidence that the neural structures implicated in ER in other populations differ in ASD either in function, size, or circuitry with other parts of the brain.[29–31] Finally, high rates of mood and anxiety disorders in the first-degree family members of children with ASD,[32,33] and conceptualization of such problems as part of the broader autism phenotype,[34] raise the possibility of an underlying genetic predisposition to ER problems in ASD also. For all of these reasons, the authors assert that it is more appropriate to consider impaired ER as inherent to ASD itself (eg, stemming from or directly related to having ASD).

Consistent with the heuristic of transdiagnostic processes proposed by Nolen-Hoeksema and Watkins,[35] ER deficits within ASD may be conceptualized as a proximal risk factor for expressed psychopathology. Poor ER is proximal in that it underlies the observed psychopathology (eg, self-injury, anxiety). Impaired ER, likewise, is influenced by distal factors such as genetic predisposition, heightened baseline physiologic arousal, and atypical neural circuitry.[36,37] The influence of these distal factors on a person's ER deficits may be strengthened by problems such as alexithymia, poor perspective taking, and inadequate response inhibition. Moderating factors then operate to influence how the impaired ER might be expressed in a given individual and at a given time (multifinality). The youngster with ASD with poor ER ability, when faced with the need to interact with others in ambiguous situations (eg, sixth grade lunch-room), might become extremely anxious or agitated.

ILLUSTRATIVE CASE EXAMPLE

Johnny is a 12-year-old boy who was diagnosed with high-functioning autism at the age of 11, based on scores above the autism cut-off on the Autism Diagnostic Interview-Revised and above the autism spectrum disorder cut-off on the Autism Diagnostic Observation Schedule. He obtained a full-scale IQ score of 90. Johnny's family history is notable for several psychiatric disorders, with 3 first-degree relatives with a depression history, 1 with bipolar disorder, 3 with anxiety disorder diagnoses, and 2 with attention-deficit/hyperactivity disorder (ADHD). Johnny's first diagnosis, at the age of 7 years, was ADHD, which was followed 6 months later by a diagnosis of bipolar disorder. Between the ages of 8 and 11 years old, he was on 23 different medications in an attempt to manage his emotions and behavior. Unfortunately, the medications, particularly those utilized as a treatment for bipolar disorder, were not effective, and he developed tics. During this period of time, he also had 3 psychiatric hospitalizations. A comprehensive assessment of his psychiatric history using the Autism Comorbidity Interview[38] at age 12 supported a past depressive disorder diagnosis but failed to confirm the presence of bipolar disorder. Specifically, there was no evidence of any mania or hypomania. It was clear, however, that problems with self-control and ER were present as a very young child. He was an irritable toddler, easily triggered and upset, per his mother's report. When upset, he would bang his head or pull his hair out. Although he did "bounce between being sad or depressed and irritable or angry," further probing revealed clear ASD-related triggers to his mood changes, such as loud, sudden noises, his schedule being changed, or a meal being late triggering a meltdown, and poor social communication skills (eg, misunderstanding sarcasm), leading to frustration. He had very poor insight into these concerns, including low scores on several self-report psychiatric screeners. His treatment plan includes a focus on increasing his self-awareness and emotion understanding, reducing the number of psychotropic medications, conducting a functional behavior assessment to identify potential antecedents to his meltdowns, addressing the identified external triggers, and teaching him ER skills.

CURRENT APPROACHES TO PRACTICE

At this time, evidence-based tools with which to accurately assess ER that have been validated in clients with ASD are lacking. In light of difficulties with insight and labeling of one's own emotions, self-report is likely to be insufficient on its own when completing the assessment and case formulation phase of treatment. Observational approaches (eg, seeing how the client responds to a mildly frustrating situation) can yield important information. It is important to assess the client's general attention to emotional states, capacity to connect to these states and describe them, and ability to differentiate among similar but unique emotions (eg, upset and angry). A thorough evaluation should also try to separate core impairments in receptive and expressive communication and social interaction from maladaptive ER. The types of regulatory strategies primarily relied on by the client, and those that may be underdeveloped, should inform treatment planning.

Although there is little controlled clinical research on the efficacy of ER-focused interventions for people with ASD, there are several plausible and potentially effective intervention approaches to consider. Drawing from the extant research on treatment of co-occurring problems, such as anxiety and mood disturbance, the predominant psychosocial approach is cognitive–behavioral therapy (CBT).[39–41] CBT-based approaches for clients with ASD often incorporate content to address ER deficits.[42,43] There is great variability in the degree to which ER training is included in such interventions, however, and evaluation of the relative import of various treatment components, including ER training, has not been conducted. Few treatment programs have been developed explicitly to improve ER ability in clients with ASD. The Exploring Feelings program[42] is a CBT-based intervention for school-aged children, with specific curricula for anxiety and for anger. It includes affect education, cognitive restructuring, and appropriate strategies to manage intense emotion. This program was recently modified for use with younger children (5–7 years) with ASD,[44] and results of an initial open trial indicated improvement in emotion lability and regulation.[45]

In light of evidence that individuals with ASD tend to engage in suppression and struggle with reappraisal, targeting increased cognitive flexibility in treatment is recommended.[23] There is empirical evidence that many of the cognitive regulatory strategies (eg, suppression, rumination) load onto a single latent factor and that these cognitive strategies are more strongly associated with psychopathology than adaptive cognitive strategies (eg, reappraisal, problem-solving).[9] Aldao and Nolen-Hoeksema[9] proposed that clients may develop a default regulatory approach that, in essence, overwhelms their ability to use newly learned, more adaptive strategies such as reappraisal. As such, treatments outside of traditional CBT, which tends to focus on restructuring of thoughts to alter feelings, may be beneficial. For example, meditation, mindfulness training, and acceptance-based approaches may help the client to reduce attempts to suppress feelings, which might enhance his or her willingness and ability to develop stronger adaptive regulatory strategies.

Psychoeducation and acceptance-based approaches may be especially helpful, given the chronic and pervasive nature of ASD. Indeed, a premise of dialectical behavior therapy (DBT[46]), a well-supported treatment for borderline personality disorder, which is characterized by extreme emotion dysregulation, is balancing acceptance of self (as is) with desire for change. Although there has been consideration of how to adapt DBT for clients with ASD,[47] there have been no clinical trials, and there is no published treatment outcome research. Mindfulness and acceptance-based approaches (MABIs), such as DBT, have been used extensively to treat problems with ER. MABIs differ from traditional CBT, primarily in how the patient's relationship to his/her feelings and thoughts is conceptualized. Rather than identification and alteration of maladaptive or incorrect thoughts and unhelpful feelings (CBT), MABIs strive to help the patient change his or her relationship with (or view of) the problem, become less fused with his or her own thoughts (accepting a thought as just a thought), and behave in a fashion consistent with his or her goals and values.[48] MABIs are associated with strong and durable improvements in symptoms of anxiety and depression and increased use of adaptive ER strategies,[49] and they have recently been shown to be as effective as CBT for treatment of anxiety.[50]

Regardless of treatment approach, a more intensive focus on developing the client's emotional awareness and ability to recognize and report on his or her emotional state is often required for clients with ASD, compared to those with other (non-ASD) diagnoses. Improving emotional insight and regulatory skills can be complicated by other treatments the client is receiving, especially medication. Between 50% and 75% of child clients with ASD are prescribed psychoactive medications,[51–53] often for target problems that might arguably be rooted in poor ER, such as irritability.[54] If a medication is dampening an emotional response, this may further complicate efforts to work on increasing emotional insight and awareness.

Often it can be helpful to use visual strategies to work on identifying, understanding, and communicating about one's own emotions. One example of a visual system that is widely used to teach these basic emotion skills is The Incredible Five Point Scale.[55] Although there has not been any systematic research on this program, it was developed based on clinical experience, was designed specifically for ASD and related populations, and has been applied across the range of intellectual and verbal abilities. In short, it provides a metric for helping the child to identify and communicate varying degrees of emotion from a scale of 1 (this never bothers me) to 5 (this could make me lose control). The skills are taught using specific situations identified by the child and/ or a caregiver or a standard set of picture cards of different situations, which the child then learns to place into a chart with pockets corresponding to 1 thru 5. The intent is that the child will learn to notice these situations, have a way to communicate about his or her emotions (eg, I am at a 3, either verbally or with picture cards), and then strategies can be taught regarding what to do in those situations. Although this is just 1 example, and it is a fairly narrow set of skills, the concepts the scale embodies (eg, incorporating visual cues, making emotion as concrete and possible, and individualizing ER interventions) are all useful approaches to consider.

Behaviors and deficits that are core to the ASD diagnosis (eg, impaired reciprocal social behavior) must be considered, and clinicians must be mindful of ASD-specific factors (both proximal and distal) that might influence ER ability. Related to this, moderators of poor ER manifestation can sometimes be managed antecedently (eg, planning for where to sit in the lunchroom). A common approach to handling problematic behavior is to complete a functional behavior analysis and, based on results, provide individualized positive behavioral supports (see also Doehring and Hagopian, this issue).[56] This approach often focuses on modifying external factors that may trigger negative emotional reactions. This type of intervention is rooted in a long history of behavioral analysis that has a wealth of support for its effectiveness dating back to the 1960s.[57] However, a limitation is that it tends to be focused on specific problems and situations and thus the impact may not generalize to other stress-provoking situations. Thus, while it is always useful to identify any environmental factors that may be exacerbating the situation, this needs to be supplemented with teaching of appropriate alternative behaviors and skills.

SUMMARY

In sum, it is important to consider ER deficits when addressing severe behavioral disturbance and situations of apparent psychiatric comorbidity in ASD. Poor regulation of emotions is likely to underlie many of the observed manifestations of both internalizing and externalizing concerns. Further, impaired ER can exacerbate problems with attention, communication, problem solving, and social interaction.[58] This article outlined many characteristics of ASD that may directly contribute to impaired ER in this population, and how ER impairment then acts as a proximal risk factor for the expression of psychopathology in clients with ASD. Unfortunately, research on ER in ASD is in its infancy. Further research is needed to better understand the specific mechanisms involved.

Measures that are sensitive to ER deficits in ASD need to be developed and validated. Accurate assessment is critical, both in terms of its role in treatment planning,[13] and in determining outcome in clinical trials. For many reasons, standard measures developed for other populations may not be clinically sensitive or appropriate for use in ASD. Standard questionnaires are often verbally loaded with items such as "complains of" that make them inapplicable to the limited and nonverbal ASD population. Further, ER problems may manifest differently in ASD.[15,38,59] Thus, in order to improve both understanding and treatment of ER problems in ASD, assessment may need to be addressed first.

Given the growing body of research implicating ER deficits in many of the psychiatric and behavioral problems manifested by clients with ASD, the authors propose that a focus on ER and its possible expression in people with ASD be considered in research on treatment development and evaluation. Although this article described some treatment strategies that incorporate ER as a component of the intervention, there is very little clinical trials research in ASD explicitly focused on ER. Further, some treatments that effectively improve ER in other populations, such as acceptance and mindfulness-based interventions, have yet to be tested in ASD. There remains a critical need to develop and study effective treatments for the range of manifestations of ER concerns in ASD. The field of affective neuroscience has much to offer in this respect. It may be possible, for instance, to develop interventions that target ER capacity directly. Doing so may have cascading benefits on multiple expressed problems (eg, irritability, anxiety). Although this type of basic and applied research is needed across the lifespan in ASD, it is notable that there have been no published ER studies of adolescents with ASD. Given that this is a developmental period characterized by a heightened risk for psychopathology and emotional reactivity,[60] hormonal and neural changes that promote cognitive flexibility and increase the saliency of social incentives (eg, peer approval),[61] and complex and often highly ambiguous social challenges that require effective regulation of emotions for successful navigation, understanding the role of ER impairment in adolescence may be a priority.

REFERENCES

1. Thompson RA. Emotion regulation: a theme in search of a definition. Monogr Soc Res Child 1994;59(2–3):25–52.
2. Gross JJ. The emerging field of emotion regulation: an integrative review. Rev Gen Psychol 1998;2(5):271–99.
3. Cole PM, Martin SE, Dennis TA. Emotion regulation as a scientific construct: methodological challenges and directions for child development research. Child Dev 2004;75(2):317–33.
4. Eisenberg N, Spinrad TL. Emotion-related regulation: sharpening the definition. Child Dev 2004;75(2):334–9.
5. Campos JJ, Frankel CB, Camras L. On the nature of emotion regulation. Child Dev 2004;75(2):377–94.

6. Siener S, Kerns KA. Emotion regulation and depressive symptoms in preadolescence. Child Psychiatry Hum Dev 2012;43(3):414–30.

7. Rieffe C, Oosterveld P, Terwogt MM, et al. Emotion regulation and internalizing symptoms in children with autism spectrum disorders. Autism 2011;15(6):655–70.

8. Cisler JM, Olatunji BO, Feldner MT, et al. Emotion regulation and the anxiety disorders: an integrative review. J Psychopathol Behav Assess 2010;32(1):68–82.

9. Aldao A, Nolen-Hoeksema S, Schweizer S. Emotion-regulation strategies across psychopathology: a meta-analytic review. Clin Psychol Rev 2010;30(2):217–37.

10. Mazefsky CA, Herrington J, Siegel M, et al. The role of emotion regulation in autism spectrum disorders. J Am Acad Child Psychiatry 2013;52(7):679–88.

11. Mazefsky CA, Pelphrey KA, Dahl RE. The need for a broader approach to emotion regulation research in autism. Child Dev Perspect 2012;6(1):92–7.

12. Konstantareas MM, Stewart K. Affect regulation and temperament in children with autism spectrum disorder. J Autism Dev Disord 2006;36(2):143–54.

13. Mazefsky CA, White SW. The role of assessment in guiding treatment planning for youth with ASD. In: Scarpa A, White S, Attwood T, editors. Promising CBT interventions for children and adolescents with high functioning ASDs. New York: Guildford Publications; 2013.

14. Mazefsky CA, Filipink R, Link J, et al. Medical evaluation and co-morbid psychiatric disorders. In: Lubetsky MJ, Handen BL, McGonigle JJ, editors. Autism spectrum disorder. New York, NY: Oxford University Press; 2011. p. 41–83.

15. Mazefsky CA, Oswald DP, Day TN, et al. ASD, a psychiatric disorder, or both? Psychiatric diagnoses in adolescents with high-functioning ASD. J Clin Child Adolesc Psychol 2012;41(4):516–23.

16. Mazefsky CA. Managing problem emotions and behaviors in children with ASD: an assessment-driven three-step approach. Perspectives Language Learning Education 2011;19:38–47.

17. Berthoz S, Hill EL. The validity of using self-reports to assess emotion regulation abilities in adults with autism spectrum disorder. Eur Psychiatry 2005;20(3):291–8.

18. Mazefsky CA, Kao J, Oswald DP. Preliminary evidence suggesting caution in the use of psychiatric self-report measures with adolescents with high-functioning autism spectrum disorders. Research in Autism Spectrum Disorders 2011; 5(1):164–74.

19. Rieffe C, Meerum Terwogt M, Kotronopoulou K. Awareness of single and multiple emotions in high-functioning children with autism. J Autism Dev Disord 2007; 37(3):455–65.

20. Ciarrochi J, Heaven PC, Supavadeeprasit S. The link between emotion identification skills and socio-emotional functioning in early adolescence: a 1-year longitudinal study. J Adolesc 2008;31(5):565–82.

21. Barrett LF, Gross J, Christensen TC, et al. Knowing what you're feeling and knowing what to do about it: mapping the relation between emotion differentiation and emotion regulation. Cogn Emot 2001;15(6):713–24.

22. Saarni C. The development of emotional competence. New York: Guilford Press/ Guilford Publications, Inc; 1999.

23. Samson AC, Huber O, Gross JJ. Emotion regulation in Asperger's syndrome and high-functioning autism. Emotion 2012;12(4):659–65.

24. Williams DL, Goldstein G, Minshew NJ. Neuropsychologic functioning in children with autism: further evidence for disordered complex information-processing. Child Neuropsychol 2006;12(4–5):279–98.

25. Baron-Cohen S. Mindblindness: an essay on autism and theory of mind. Palatino (CA): MIT press; 1997.

26. Murray MJ. Attention-deficit/hyperactivity disorder in the context of autism spectrum disorders. Curr Psychiatry Rep 2010;12(5):382–8.
27. Dunn W, City K. The impact of sensory processing abilities on the daily lives of young children and their families: a conceptual model. Infants Young Child 1997;9(4):24–35.
28. Rogers SJ, Ozonoff S. Annotation: what do we know about sensory dysfunction in autism? A critical review of the empirical evidence. J Child Psychol Psychiatry 2005;46(12):1255–68.
29. Monk CS. The development of emotion-related neural circuitry in health and psychopathology. Dev Psychopathol 2008;20(4):1231–50.
30. Herrington JD, Schultz R. Neuroimaging of developmental disorders. In: Shenton ME, Turetsky BI, editors. Understanding neuropsychiatric disorders: insights from neuroimaging. Cambridge (United Kingdom): Cambridge University Press; 2010. p. 517–36.
31. Mazefsky CA, Minshew NJ. Clinical pearl: the spectrum of autism-from neuronal connections to behavioral expression. Virtual Mentor 2010;12(11):867–72.
32. Mazefsky CA, Folstein SE, Lainhart JE. Overrepresentation of mood and anxiety disorders in adults with autism and their first-degree relatives: what does it mean? Autism Res 2008;1(3):193–7.
33. Mazefsky CA, Conner CM, Oswald DP. Association between depression and anxiety in high-functioning children with autism spectrum disorders and maternal mood symptoms. Autism Res 2010;3(3):120–7.
34. Gerdts J, Bernier R. The broader autism phenotype and its implications on the etiology and treatment of autism spectrum disorders. Autism Res Treat 2011; 2011:1–18.
35. Nolen-Hoeksema S, Watkins ER. A heuristic for developing transdiagnostic models of psychopathology: explaining multifinality and divergent trajectories. Perspect Psychol Sci 2011;6(6):589–609.
36. Nummenmaa L, Engell AD, Von dem Hagen E, et al. Autism spectrum traits predict the neural response to eye gaze in typical individuals. Neuroimage 2012; 59(4):3356–63.
37. Redcay E. The superior temporal sulcus performs a common function for social and speech perception: implications for the emergence of autism. Neurosci Biobehav Rev 2008;32(1):123–42.
38. Leyfer OT, Folstein SE, Bacalman S, et al. Comorbid psychiatric disorders in children with autism: interview development and rates of disorders. J Autism Dev Disord 2006;36(7):849–61.
39. Lang R, Regester A, Lauderdale S, et al. Treatment of anxiety in autism spectrum disorders using cognitive behaviour therapy: a systematic review. Dev Neurorehabil 2010;13(1):53–63.
40. Lickel A, Maclean WE, Hepburn AB. Assessment of the prerequisite skills for cognitive behavioral therapy in children with and without autism spectrum disorders. J Autism Dev Disord 2012;42:992–1000.
41. Scarpa A, White SW, Attwood T, editors. Cognitive-behavioral interventions for children and adolescents with high-functioning autism spectrum disorders. New York: Guildford Publications; 2013.
42. Attwood T. Cognitive behaviour therapy for children and adults with Asperger's syndrome. Behav Change 2004;21(3):147–61.
43. Reaven J, Blakeley-Smith A, Culhane-Shelburne K, et al. Group cognitive behavior therapy for children with high-functioning autism spectrum disorders and anxiety: a randomized trial. J Child Psychol Psychiatry 2012;53(4):410–9.

44. Scarpa A, Wells A, Attwood T. Exploring feelings for young children with high-functioning Autism or Asperger's disorder. London: Jessica Kingsley Publishers; 2013.

45. Scarpa A, Reyes NM. Improving emotion regulation with CBT in young children with high functioning autism spectrum disorders: a pilot study. Behav Cogn Psychother 2011;39(4):495–500.

46. Linehan MM. Cognitive-behavioral treatment of borderline personality disorder. New York, NY: Guilford Press/Guilford Publications, Inc; 1993.

47. Hartmann K, Urbano M, Manser K, et al. Modified dialectical behavior therapy to improve emotion regulation in autism spectrum disorders. In: Richardson C, Wood R, editors. Autism spectrum disorders. Hauppauge, NY: Nova Science Publishers; 2012. p. 41–72.

48. Vøllestad J, Nielsen MB, Nielsen GH. Mindfulness- and acceptance-based interventions for anxiety disorders: a systematic review and meta-analysis. Br J Clin Psychol 2012;51(3):239–60.

49. Kumar S, Feldman G, Hayes A. Changes in mindfulness and emotion regulation in an exposure-based cognitive therapy for depression. Cognit Ther Res 2008; 32(6):734–44.

50. Arch JJ, Eifert GH, Davies C, et al. Randomized clinical trial of cognitive behavioral therapy (CBT) versus acceptance and commitment therapy (ACT) for mixed anxiety disorders. J Consult Clin Psychol 2012;80(5):750–65.

51. Aman MG, Lam KS, Van Bourgondien ME. Medication patterns in patients with autism: temporal, regional, and demographic influences. J Child Adolesc Psychopharmacol 2005;15(1):116–26.

52. Oswald DP, Sonenklar NA. Medication use among children with autism spectrum disorders. J Child Adolesc Psychopharmacol 2007;17(3):348–55.

53. Siegel M. Psychopharmacology of autism spectrum disorder: evidence and practice. Child Adolesc Psychiatr Clin N Am 2012;21(4):957–73.

54. Williamson ED, Martin A. Psychotropic medications in autism: practical considerations for parents. J Autism Dev Disord 2012;42(6):1249–55.

55. Buron KD, Curtis M. The incredible 5-point scale: assisting students with autism spectrum disorders in understanding social interactions and controlling their emotional responses. Shawnee Mission (KS): Autism Asperger Publishing Company; 2003.

56. Mazefsky CA, Handen BL. Addressing behavioral and emotional challenges in school-aged children with ASD. In: Lubetsky M, McGonigle J, Handen B, editors. Autism spectrum disorder. New York, NY: Oxford University Press; 2011. p. 253–69.

57. Iwata BA, Dorsey MF, Slifer KJ, et al. Toward a functional analysis of self-injury. J Appl Behav Anal 1994;27(2):197–209.

58. Laurent AC, Otr L, Rubin E. Challenges in emotional regulation in Asperger syndrome and high-functioning autism. Topics in Language Disorders 2004;4(24): 286–97.

59. Magnuson KM, Constantino JN. Characterization of depression in children with autism spectrum disorders. J Dev Behav Pediatr 2011;32:332–40.

60. Dahl RE, Gunnar MR. Heightened stress responsiveness and emotional reactivity during pubertal maturation: implications for psychopathology. Dev Psychopathol 2009;21(1):1–6.

61. Crone EA, Dahl RE. Understanding adolescence as a period of social-affective engagement and goal flexibility. Nat Rev Neurosci 2012;13(9):636–50.

Behavioral Approaches to Managing Severe Problem Behaviors in Children with Autism Spectrum and Related Developmental Disorders
A Descriptive Analysis

Peter Doehring, PhD[a],*, Brian Reichow, PhD, BCBA-D[b],
Tamara Palka, MD[c], Cara Phillips, PhD, BCBA[d], Louis Hagopian, PhD[e]

KEYWORDS

- Autism • Intellectual disability • Aggression • Self-injury • Behavioral intervention
- Applied behavior analysis • Outcome research • Children

KEY POINTS

- Severe problem behaviors such as aggression and self-injury are not uncommon in children with autism spectrum disorder (ASD) or intellectual disability (ID).
- This review covers 101 outcome studies published since 1995 that used behavioral techniques to address severe aggression, self-injury, and property destruction, in children between 6 and 18 years of age.
- Researchers relied on proactive and preventative behavioral techniques driven by functional behavioral assessment, with specific interventions associated with specific behavioral targets and functions.
- Researchers are increasingly interested in applying these techniques outside of specialized hospital and residential programs, although these techniques will be challenging for community-based practitioners to implement.

Funding Sources: Nil.
Conflicts of Interest: Nil.
The protocol for this review is registered with PROSPERO (CRD42013003105).
[a] ASD Roadmap, 5 Nine Gates Road, Chadds Ford, PA 19317, USA; [b] Child Study Center, Yale School of Medicine, 230 South Frontage Road, New Haven, CT 06519, USA; [c] Developmental Disorders Unit, Foundations Behavioral Health, 833 East Butler Avenue, Doylestown, PA 18901, USA; [d] Neurobehavioral Inpatient Unit, Kennedy Krieger Institute, The Johns Hopkins School of Medicine, 707 North Broadway, Baltimore, MD 21205, USA; [e] Neurobehavioral Inpatient Unit, Department of Psychiatry and Behavioral Sciences, Johns Hopkins University School of Medicine, The Johns Hopkins School of Medicine, 707 North Broadway, Baltimore, MD 21205, USA
* Corresponding author.
E-mail address: peter@asdroadmap.org

Child Adolesc Psychiatric Clin N Am 23 (2014) 25–40
http://dx.doi.org/10.1016/j.chc.2013.08.001
1056-4993/14/$ – see front matter © 2014 Elsevier Inc. All rights reserved.
childpsych.theclinics.com

INTRODUCTION

The term "problem behavior" or "challenging behavior" is generally used to refer to behaviors such as aggression, self-injury, property destruction, pica, elopement, and other behaviors that can result in injury to self or others, or that can significantly impair functioning. The prevalence of behavior problems among persons with autism spectrum disorders (ASD) and related developmental disorders such as intellectual disability (ID) is approximately 50%.[1–5] Known risk factors include the severity of autistic symptoms, impulsivity, level of intellectual disability, and communication deficits.[6,7] Individuals typically display multiple types of problem behavior, and the levels of severity can range from relatively minor and short-lived to severe, chronic, and potentially life-threatening.[3,8]

The impact of such behaviors can vary from child to child. Self-injurious behavior (SIB) and aggression can lead to significant injuries to self and others.[9–12] Problem behavior can severely limit the integration of the person into their school and community, and place tremendous stress on the family.[13,14] Children with ASD are 9 times more likely to seek emergency-room care related to mental health issues[15] and, in some cases, may require acute psychiatric hospitalization.[16] In a recent survey commissioned by the Pennsylvania Bureau of Autism Services,[17] almost 9% of Pennsylvania families with children with ASD in middle or high school reported that they had sought urgent hospital care (eg, emergency-room use or hospitalization) in the past year, most often for aggression or self-injury. Individuals with persistent problem behavior are at increased risk for residential placement, seclusion, physical restraint, other restrictive measures, and excessive medication.[9,18] The increasing rates of ASD,[19] coupled with the high prevalence of problem behavior, and its adverse impact on children and families, makes this a topic of major concern.

Fortunately, a range of therapeutic interventions designed to address problem behavior associated with ASD have been and are being developed. Although no medication can address the core deficits in ASD at present, they are used to treat psychiatric conditions that may co-occur with ASD and to target associated features such as irritability and problem behavior,[20] and thus better enable individuals with ASD to participate in therapeutic programming.[21] At present only 2 medications, risperidone and aripiprazole, are approved by the Food and Drug Administration for addressing irritability in children with ASD. However, other medications have shown promise, and their safety and efficacy is currently being evaluated.[22,23]

Behavioral interventions based on applied behavior analysis (ABA) relevant to ASD can broadly be categorized as either comprehensive or problem-focused. Comprehensive interventions, including early intensive behavioral intervention, use behavioral intervention tactics to intensively teach a broad range of adaptive skills over an extended period. These methods are generally regarded as empirically supported,[24] but are not the focus of this review. Rather, this article focuses on problem-focused behavioral interventions that are more time-limited and are designed to address problem behavior such as aggression and self-injury. Studies describing this category of behavioral interventions for aggression, self-injury, and related behaviors span a period of 40 years.[11,25–29] Contemporary behavioral interventions use a range of behavioral procedures based on the results of functional behavioral assessment, which is designed to identify the controlling antecedents and reinforcing consequences for problem behavior. Research shows that, in 60% to 75% of cases, problem behavior is maintained by social consequences, most commonly attention, access to preferred materials, and escape from instruction.[30–32] Interventions based on the results of a functional analysis are viewed as more proactive because they aim to prevent the occurrence of problem behaviors, and place more emphasis on targeted adaptive skills including communication, social, and leisure skills. With the widespread use of functional-based interventions, there has been decreased use of punishment.[11] Although punishment and other reactive strategies (eg, blocking behavior, or using protective devices such as helmets or arm-splints to physically inhibit or prevent self-injury) are used with decreasing frequency, these procedures may be necessary as a last resort in the most severe and treatment-resistant cases.[33] However, it may be difficult or impossible to use reactive strategies that are relatively more intrusive and restrictive outside of highly specialized settings. A more detailed description of behavioral assessment and treatment procedures for severe problem behavior is beyond the scope of the current review, and a more in-depth discussion of these procedures and their integrated use with pharmacologic interventions can be found elsewhere.[34]

Several reviewers have sought to identify the most effective interventions for problem behaviors. Most of these reviews are either limited in scope[35] or rely on a more traditional, somewhat subjective selection and analysis of the available literature. Thus, they may capitalize on the reviewer's particular experience or perspective but offer no guarantee that the review is comprehensive, or that results derived from high-quality outcome research have been appropriately weighted. More recent reviews involve systematically subjecting the available outcome research to a more rigorous analysis, whereby the quality of individual outcome studies focused on a specific method or target is first objectively assessed, after which those studies achieving an established standard are evaluated as a group to determine if there are sufficient data to conclude that the practice is evidence based. Such reviews have identified several interventions for problem behaviors in children with ASD that are evidence based, especially those derived from ABA that design treatments based on a functional behavioral assessment.[36–38]

At the same time, there has been an increasing interest in helping community-based clinicians apply research findings to the care of children in their day-to-day practice. For example, the National Autism Center[38] sought to break down recommendations according to the diagnosis of the child and the broad category of target behavior or skill. The National Professional Development Center[36] developed a range of supporting materials, including evidence-based practice briefs and fidelity checklists. It is less clear, however, whether the assessment and intervention protocols for severe problem behaviors described by researchers can be replicated by community-based practitioners (eg, via school-based or outpatient programs). In the case of severe problem behavior, the successful replication of these strategies may help to reduce the reliance on expensive residential or inpatient treatment options, perhaps by building the capacity to more quickly identify and effectively address problem behavior before it becomes a crisis. This potential may now be greater than ever, given that schools are now mandated to implement behavior support plans when behavior problems linked to a child's disability result in suspension or expulsion, and given that some of the autism insurance legislation passed in the past 5 years has emphasized the role of behavior analysis.

The goal of this article is to evaluate outcome research that has used behavioral interventions to decrease severe problem behaviors among children and adolescents with ASD and related disabilities, preparatory to a more formal evaluation addressing the quality of research. The following questions guided this review:

- What kinds of behaviors have researchers targeted?
- What individual interventions or combinations of interventions have been considered, and how effective have these been in decreasing severe problem behaviors?
- Are there differences in terms of the kinds of interventions used, either alone or in various combinations, under different conditions?
- What other support (eg, assessment procedures, efforts to increase fidelity) is used with these interventions?
- Are there patterns in the use of interventions under these different conditions that suggest how best to translate these research findings into practice?

METHOD
Study-Selection Criteria

Studies included in the review meet the following inclusion criteria. First, the study involved children ages 6 to 18 years with ID and/or ASD. Individual participants meeting the criteria were included from studies in which only some participants fell within the 6- to 18-year age span, so far as results for each of the individuals could be distinguished from one another. Second, the study used an experimental design, including randomized controlled trial, quasi-experimental multiple-group comparison, or single-subject experimental design, with enough replications to judge the presence of a functional relation. Third, the study involved a behavioral intervention to decrease severe aggression, self-injury, or property destruction. Finally, the study must have been published in English in a peer-reviewed journal between 1995 and 2012, and listed in online databases by October 2012. Though designed to be replicable and comprehensive, the search was not expected to identify every study on this topic. Nonetheless, a sufficient number of studies were identified to consider them to be representative of the literature.

Search Methods and Study Selection

The authors conducted an electronic database search of Medline and PsycINFO in October 2012 using a strategy including key terms for the population (ie, "autis,*" "intellectual disabilit,*" "developmental disabilit,*" or "mental retard*") and for the target behavior (ie, "aggress,*" "self-injur,*" or "destruct*") anywhere in the text of the record. The searches were then combined for the population and target behavior to form a pool of potential studies for abstract screening. Two study authors (P.D., T.P.) independently conducted abstract screening using the diagnosis, age, type of problem behavior, behavior severity, and article type, and identified 199 potential studies meriting more thorough screening. These 2 researchers independently conducted a screening of the entire article, using the same criteria, and identified 101 of the 199 articles that met all inclusion criteria. Full reviews were independently conducted by 1 of several study authors (P.D., B.R., L.H., C.P.) using the variables described below (a complete list of articles reviewed is available from the first author on request). Articles were allocated to reviewers for screening and review, with an overlap of 20% to allow calculation of interrater reliability. Interrater reliability for abstract screening was 96% and for article screening was 89%. Interrater reliability for coding of the full review ranged from 80% to 97%, with an average interrater reliability of 87%.

Variable Definitions and Coding

Participants

With respect to *Age Group*, the review distinguished between school-aged children (6–12 years old) and adolescents (13–18 years old).

With respect to *Diagnosis*, participants were categorized as having ASD, ID, or both.

For those with ID, their *Level* of ID was coded as Borderline/Mild (eg, IQ 60–80), Moderate (eg, IQ 40–60), or Severe (eg, IQ less than 40).

Finally, the *Setting* in which treatment was provided to the participant was noted, distinguishing between inpatient, residential, and other programs (eg, in the home or school).

Behavior

Distinction was made between different *Types* of behavior target (aggression, self-injury, destruction, or combined targets addressing 2 or more of the above). When deciding which outcome studies to include in the analyses, the following were considered to be evidence of *Severity*: (1) the behavior was specifically labeled as severe, intense, or using a similar term; (2) the behavior resulted in injuries; (3) the behavior triggered the use of restrictive interventions (eg, seclusion or restraint) or protective equipment (eg, helmets, arm splints); or (4) the child was served in a restrictive setting (eg, inpatient program or residential program), regardless of whether the behavior was cited as a reason for the placement. The *Function* of the behavior was also categorized (Attention, Automatic, Escape, Sensory, Tangible, Unspecified, Multiply Determined, or Other).

Interventions

To code *Interventions*, the authors drew initially from the categories and definitions developed by the National Professional Development Center (NPDC) on Autism,[36] and those expected to be used to address problem behaviors: Antecedent-Based Intervention (including enriching the environment, using highly preferred activities, changing the task, and so forth), Differential Reinforcement, Extinction, Functional Communication Training, Prompting, Other Reinforcement, Response Interruption/Redirection, Self-Management, Social Narratives, Time Delay, and Other Interventions (some definitions were expanded on: Competing Stimuli was added to Antecedent Interventions, Blocking and Protective Equipment to Response Interruption, and Noncontingent Reinforcement to Reinforcement). In subsequent analyses, these were categorized as Proactive Strategies and Reactive Strategies (**Table 1**). Whenever possible, the authors sought to broadly categorize participants with respect to their reported *Response to Treatment* as Responders (ie, 80% or greater reduction in problem behavior relative to baseline levels across conditions), Partial Responders (25%–75% Reduction), Mixed (less than 25% Reduction), Negative, or Response Could Not Be Determined. Reductions were established relative to a baseline that was determined to be valid according to the standard of Reichow and colleagues.[39] At the completion of coding, studies using Other Interventions were reviewed to identify other categories. The categories of Punishment (including time-out, response cost, and so forth) and Sensory Integration were added.

Other study characteristics

It was noted whether *Behavioral Assessment* relied on observations, interview of caregivers or others, formal checklists, and/or analog functional analysis (eg, involving the use of controlled conditions whereby antecedent and consequent variables of interest are systematically manipulated and behavior is directly observed). With respect to *Diagnostic Assessment* for participants identified with an ASD, whether specific

Table 1
Number of participant-intervention combinations by target behavior, function, response to treatment, treatment used, and setting

Interventions	Target Behavior		Function				Response		Treatment Used		Setting		
	Aggression	Self-Injury	Attention	Automatic	Escape	Tangible	Responder	Mixed	Alone	Combination	Inpatient	Residential	Other
Proactive													
Antecedent	11	27++	9	10	24	11	28	30	25+	33	32	10	16
DRO	13+	12	22	5	24	20	43+	7-	22+	28	26	2	22+
FCT	14++	5	20	2	21	9	19	21	11	29	23	8	9
Reinforcement	5	7	11	4	5	8	12	12	4	20	18	2	4
Reactive													
Extinction	13+	11	16	4	18	11	19	20	0--	39+	26	7	6
Punishment	5	4	5	4	6	4	10	4	3	11	10	3	1
Resp. Inter.	3	16++	4	7++	6	3	16	8	5	19	13	4	7
Total	64	82	53	21	59	37	147	102	70	179	148	36	65

Z-score greater than expected: +P<.05; ++P<.01; Z-score less than expected: -P<.05; --P<.01.
Abbreviations: DRO, differential reinforcement of other behavior; FCT, functional communication training; Resp. Inter., response interruption.

information was cited in support of the diagnosis was noted. With respect to *Cognitive Assessment* for participants identified with ID, whether the assessor was identified, or the results of any assessments were cited was noted. Other factors to be noted were: the publication *Period* (1995–2003 or 2004–2012); whether a group design (GD) or single-subject experimental design (SSD) was used; whether measures were taken to increase *Fidelity* (eg, the use of treatment manuals, detailed descriptions of training, or actual measurement of treatment fidelity); and the *Periodical* in which the findings were published.

RESULTS
General Study Characteristics

Settings
Of the identified studies, more were published between 1995 and 2003 (65) than during the period between 2004 and 2012 (39). Most of the studies (ie, 76%) were conducted in the context of relatively more restrictive settings (eg, inpatient or residential programs) as opposed to other programs (eg, home or school). To prepare data for chi-square (χ^2) analysis, the authors categorized studies that were conducted across multiple settings using the least restrictive setting: that is, a study conducted in a residential program and in the home was categorized under Other Program. A χ^2 test of the interaction of time period and setting was significant (df = 2, $P<.05$), revealing that a significantly higher than expected number of the identified studies were conducted in the home or school in the later time period (**Table 2**).

Periodical
Half (50%) of the 101 studies were reported in the *Journal of Applied Behavior Analysis*, a smaller proportion were reported in *Behavioral Intervention* and *Research in Developmental Disabilities* (17% and 11%, respectively), and the rest were scattered across a dozen other journals.

Fidelity
Almost all (93%) of the studies relied on detailed descriptions of intervention while relatively few (14%) included measures of fidelity, and only 2 made use of a manual.

Assessment
Analog functional analysis was the behavioral assessment method used in the majority (78%) of studies. The remaining studies relied primarily on less structured observations (18%), interviews (12%), or checklists (4%). Fewer than 10% of the studies provided any additional information, however, regarding cognitive or diagnostic assessment. All of the identified studies used SSD to evaluate interventions, which allowed for demonstration of control through the replication of treatment effects.

Table 2
Number of studies by setting and period

Period	Inpatient	Residential	Other	Total
1995–2003	43	10	10	63
2004–2012	18	5	15[+]	38
Total	61	15	25	101

Z-score greater than expected: [+]$P<.05$.

Participants

Some studies included multiple participants (a total of 150 across the 101 studies), therefore all analyses of the participants' characteristics were conducted at the level of the participant and not the study.

Age and gender

The majority of the participants were school-aged children (98; 65%), and more than 70% (102) were male. χ^2 tests did not reveal any interactions between the time period studied and either the age group or the gender of the participant.

ASD and ID

The vast majority of participants (137 of 150; 91%) likely had ID, with more than one-half (78; 57%) having severe to profound ID. Almost half (72 of 150; 48%) had ASD. Less than one-half (59; 43%) with ID also had ASD, while most of those with ASD also had ID (59 of 72; 83%). A χ^2 test did not reveal any significant interactions between the level of ID and either the presence of ASD or the time period. Among participants with ID, a significant χ^2 (df $= 1$, $P<.001$) for the interaction between the time period and the presence of ASD revealed that the number of participants with ASD in studies published between 2004 and 2012 was significantly higher than expected ($Z = 2.23$, $P<.05$). Whereas the number of participants with ID dropped markedly from the earlier to the more recent time period (from 64 to 14), the decrease from the earlier to the more recent time period was much less marked for those participants with ID and ASD (from 32 to 27).

Behavior Targets, Interventions, and Outcomes

Behavioral targets

Simple analyses of behavior targets, interventions, and outcomes were conducted at the level of the participant. Self-injury was the most common single behavior targeted (53 of 150 participants, or 35%), followed by aggression (40 participants; 27%) and property destruction (5 participants; 3%). Combined behaviors were addressed in 52 participants (35%).

Evidence that problem behavior was severe

The majority (114 participants, or 76%) met criteria as having severe problem behavior based on their placement in a hospital or residential program. Problem behavior was explicitly labeled as severe for 98 participants (65%), resulted in injuries in 68 participants (45%), and required the use of seclusion, restraint, or protective equipment in 29 participants (19%). For many participants (99; 66%), multiple factors were cited as evidence of severe problem behavior, and in only 6 participants was the problem behavior determined to be severe solely by virtue of the child's residential placement.

Behavioral function

Escape was identified as the function in 59 participants (39%) and attention in 50 participants (33%), followed by tangibles (37), automatic (21), and sensory (6). Multiple functions were identified in 40 participants (27%), and only 1 study did not report the use of any form of functional behavior assessment.

Response to treatment

The majority of participants (98; 65%) were characterized as responders, which was defined as those for whom an 80% or greater reduction in problem behavior was achieved, relative to baseline. Thirty-one (21%) were characterized as partial responders (25%–79% reduction) while relatively few participants (19; 13%) were characterized as nonresponders in that their outcomes were mixed, negative, or could not be determined.

Type of interventions
The most frequently used interventions were antecedent interventions (in 58, or 40% of participants), and differential reinforcement (50; 34% of participants); these were followed closely by extinction and functional communication training, used with 39 and 40 participants, respectively (27% each). Other reinforcement (primarily noncontingent reinforcement) and response interruption were each used in 24 participants (16%). Punishment or other forms of intervention were used in 14 participants. Almost all cases (97%) used at least 1 of the 7 interventions identified herein. Many of these (52%) used combinations of these interventions, with an average of 1.8 interventions per case. Other categories of interventions were used less than 5% of the time (eg, self-management, sensory integration, social narratives, and time delay) while other interventions that could not be classified were used in 14 participants (or 11%). Subsequent analyses focused on the 7 remaining categories grouped as proactive strategies (antecedent interventions, differential reinforcement, functional communication training, and other reinforcement) and reactive strategies (extinction, punishment, or response interruption).

Interactions Between Behavior Interventions and Other Factors

Because many of the cases entailed the use of multiple interventions, analyses of the interactions of interventions with other variables are based on up to 249 participant-intervention combinations noted among the participants and studies reviewed. These results are unlikely to be skewed by any specific participant, because only 4 cases used more than 3 of the 7 interventions listed herein.

Combinations of interventions
The authors considered whether certain interventions were more likely to be used alone or in combination with one another. A χ^2 test revealed significant variability (df = 6, $P<.001$), reflecting that in the 58 cases in which antecedent intervention was used, it was used alone more often than expected (in 25 or 43% of these). Differential reinforcement was also used alone more often than expected (in 22 out of 50 participants, or 44%), and extinction was used exclusively in combination with other interventions (see **Table 1**). It was also considered whether specific combinations of interventions were more likely than others to emerge. The most prevalent combinations of interventions were functional communication training with extinction (19 participants) followed by antecedent interventions and extinction (14 participants). Formal tests of significance could not be applied, however, because of the large number of cells with low frequencies.

Interactions with behavioral targets
The authors considered whether different kinds of interventions were used to address specific and prevalent behavior targets. These analyses focused on aggression and self-injury, and excluded participants for whom property destruction or combined behaviors were targeted. A χ^2 test revealed significant variations in the distribution of interventions as a function of behavior target (df = 6, $P<.001$). Antecedent interventions and response interruption were much more likely to be used to address self-injury, whereas differential reinforcement, functional communication, and extinction were more commonly used to target aggression (see **Table 1**).

Interactions with behavior functions

It was considered whether different interventions were used to address specific and prevalent behavior functions. The analysis therefore focused on targets with a single identified attention, automatic, escape, or tangible function, and excluded infrequent functions (eg, sensory) and multiple functions; this yielded a total of 170 participant-intervention combinations. A χ^2 test revealed a significant interaction of intervention and function (df = 18, P = <.05), such that the use of response interruption in response to behavior serving an automatic function was higher than expected (see **Table 1**).

Interactions between response to treatment and interventions

To increase the power to detect differences in the response to treatment, a distinction was made between responders and all other categories, collapsing partial responders and nonresponders into a mixed responder category. Significant differences in the response to treatment were noted (df = 6, P<.001), reflecting that differential reinforcement was associated with a strong response to treatment and was not associated with a mixed response to treatment (see **Table 1**).

Interactions with other participant and setting variables

A χ^2 test revealed a trend toward an uneven distribution of interventions across settings (df = 12, P<.10), such that differential reinforcement was more likely to be used in other settings (see **Table 1**). Otherwise, no patterns were noted in the distribution of interventions as a function of the presence of ASD, the level of ID, or the time period when the study was published.

DISCUSSION

In this review of more than 100 peer-reviewed studies involving 150 children and adolescents, the authors sought to characterize outcome research assessing the impact of behavioral interventions on severe self-injury, aggression, and related behaviors in young people with ASD and/or ID. Severe problem behavior was defined as those behaviors that have resulted either in injury, specialized placement, or restrictive interventions. Most participants were treated in specialized settings, nearly half had caused injuries to themselves or others, and two-thirds met criteria as having "severe" behavior for multiple reasons, suggesting that this literature describes a very challenging population that is at extreme risk. Although the difficulties these children and their families face are sobering, the results of this review are encouraging. In short, it reveals that there is a rich literature describing a variety of behavioral interventions that are generally effective, and increasingly applicable in a broader range of settings. More than 86% of individuals benefited from treatment, with 65% being characterized as "responders" in that their problem behavior was reduced by more than 80%. It bears noting that these outcomes should be interpreted with some caution, as they represent the outcomes of published studies subject to the inherent bias for journals to publish studies that show effects. The threshold chosen for positive response, greater than 80% reduction, was also significantly greater than thresholds typically chosen in pharmaceutical trials.[40] Another noteworthy issue is that these interventions require specialized behavioral assessment techniques, and complex and staff-intensive interventions. Thus, challenges remain in the development of the capacity to help children, families, and practitioners struggling with these behaviors. The findings also reveal patterns in the interventions used to address specific targets and functions, and set the stage for a more systematic and in-depth evaluation of the quality of the evidence. Each of these points is addressed here.

First, the significant increase over time in the number of studies reporting the successful use of these interventions in home and school settings suggests that behavioral interventions are increasingly applicable outside of specialized settings. Although the presence of severe problem behavior can be dangerous, it is also debilitating when it interferes with community integration and participation. The increase in the number of studies reporting on the treatment of severe problem behavior in community settings is therefore encouraging in that it suggests that individuals do not necessarily require specialized placement to receive appropriate treatment.

Although community-based treatment has its advantages, replicating complex interventions in such settings will be challenging. The fact that very few of the reviewed studies relied on manuals or formal assessments of fidelity suggest that tools to support implementation in community settings may still need to be developed. Because these researchers sought to describe advanced behavior intervention strategies, they may sometimes have failed to describe more fundamental strategies important to successful intervention. This aspect may explain why extinction was not found to be paired more reliably with differential reinforcement or other interventions. Few studies provided much detail regarding diagnostic or cognitive assessment, suggesting that such information may be less immediately relevant to the task of developing plans to address severe aggression and self-injury. Moreover, the reality that such assessments designed originally for typically developing individuals may not yield stable and reliable results for children in behavioral crisis. The existing literature, however, does not permit us to address this question.

The approaches studied also reinforce the predominant model of behavioral intervention, which emphasizes proactive strategies, informed by functional assessment and adjusted through careful tracking of the individual child's progress. The studies reviewed describe a variety of interventions, most commonly antecedent interventions, reinforcement-based strategies, functional communication training, and extinction. These interventions not only address the immediate contextual variables that occasion and maintain problem behavior; they also establish and strengthen communication, social, and leisure skills, and so are especially relevant to children with ID. Deficits in adaptive behavior have long been identified as risk factors for problem behavior, so it is not surprising that one-half of participants had severe or profound ID, even though such levels of ID are relatively uncommon. Indeed, these interventions were just as likely to be used in children with ID regardless of whether they also had ASD. Such interventions also lend themselves to implementation in a wide range of community-based settings in some form, and with the right training and support.

These results may also suggest some specific circumstances under which certain interventions should be considered. The observations that differential reinforcement was frequently used as the sole intervention, was more likely to be studied in home and school settings, and yielded the strongest response to treatment, suggest that differential reinforcement may initially be the primary focus of intervention. The finding that antecedent intervention was often used as the sole intervention, yielded a strong response to treatment in almost 50% of cases, and was especially likely to be used to address self-injury may suggest that it be initially considered when addressing self-injury. Given that extinction was never used as the sole intervention, the authors conclude that simply ignoring severe problem behaviors in the absence of reinforcement is not consistent with current research or practices. The frequent use of response interruption to target self-injury is not surprising given the immediate risks, and this was especially true when addressing the internal and ambiguous sources of motivation for behaviors serving an automatic function. By contrast, differential reinforcement, functional communication, and extinction were more commonly used to target aggression. It was also interesting that functional communication training was accompanied by extinction more than half of the time.

A specific barrier to translating these findings into everyday practice is the complexity of the assessment process, and the implication that some settings will have to retool. For example, these findings suggest that more settings seeking to address complex and/or severe problem behaviors should probably develop the capacity to conduct more intensive and specialized functional analysis. Indeed, almost 40% of cases identified either multiple functions or an automatic function, and many instances were noted whereby functional analysis was itself adapted based on the particular responses of the child. In many cases, tailoring the intervention to the individual child also involved more than just addressing the underlying function; also noted were antecedent interventions based on competing stimulus assessment, schedules of differential reinforcement adjusted to the child's response, and noncontingent reinforcement that only worked if it involved specific reinforcers, among others. Sometimes the combinations of interventions emerged through an iterative process following very careful progress monitoring, which may underscore the need for ongoing support from professionals experienced in behavioral analysis.

There is also concern that interest in these important issues may be waning. Even during a period when the number of studies involving persons with ASD was increasing overall,[41] fewer outcome studies addressing severe aggression and self-injury, and especially for those with ID uncomplicated by ASD, were found. The authors are confident that their search strategies captured the vast majority of outcome research involving children whose severe behavior resulted in hospitalization or repeated injury, while recognizing that studies of children not in residential or hospital placements may have been missed if the study investigators did not adequately convey the severity of the behavior. Even in this case, the search would have only missed more studies from the more recent time period if there had been a significant shift in the use of the key descriptors in electronic databases. The fact that one-half of the literature reviewed here was published in a single periodical (*Journal of Applied Behavior Analysis*) may also leave the field more vulnerable to shifts in publication policy.

Because this is not a survey of actual populations or interventions as used in day-to-day practice but is a review of outcome research, these findings may be qualified in other important ways, especially as one looks toward broader implementation. On the one hand, programs that conduct research often offer more extensive staff training, maintain higher staffing ratios, and keep abreast of changes in practice. One would expect that this improves individualized treatment planning and progress monitoring, as well as fidelity of implementation. On the other hand, programs focused on practice can be developed more quickly, may have greater flexibility to partner with other community agencies, and, in the case of publicly funded services, may be motivated to develop services accessible to traditionally underserved populations. These findings suggest that the most effective collaborations leverage the expertise of centers that conduct research, to help publicly funded programs provide more specialized services.[42]

This review can only describe patterns of findings because it was not formally established that these practices are evidence based: that is, rigorous standards were not systematically applied to each outcome study, and whether there are enough studies meeting these standards that also demonstrate similar findings was not verified.[36,38,43] Nonetheless, this review confirms that there may be enough outcome research to develop precise, evidence-based practice recommendations: for example, recommending specific intervention(s) for a specific target behavior when addressing a specific behavioral function.[35,44] Such an approach would complement other kinds of systematic approaches, such as meta-analyses,[45] which focus more on patterns in reported effect sizes than on the strength of the research design per se.

Other avenues might also be explored in future reviews. Extending the review to include adults and preschoolers or less severe problem behavior would widen the application of the results, and likely double the number of studies included. Parallel reviews of other common interventions, such as psychopharmacology, may help develop more comprehensive practice guidelines. Co-occurring neurologic conditions (eg, seizure disorders), medical conditions (eg, sources of acute or chronic pain or discomfort), and other behavioral conditions (eg, sleep disorders) can also complicate individual treatment, and researchers should explore the role played by the interaction of these factors in the genesis of severe aggression and self-injury. The authors acknowledge that the bias against publication of negative findings makes it difficult to identify treatments as ineffective. An alternative encountered in this review is the systematic comparison of 2 strategies within the same participant: in this case, Devlin and colleagues[46,47] found that sensory integration treatment was much less effective in the treatment of severe problem behaviors when compared with behavioral approaches.

These results frame larger issues for professionals and policy makers seeking to help children with severe problem behaviors. In the authors' experience such behaviors often develop slowly, after opportunities are missed to address less severe behaviors through simple, positive, and preventive interventions applied systematically and intensively by community-based practitioners. The resulting deterioration in behavior is sadly predictable: caregivers and practitioners focus on managing outbursts instead of preventing them, until a crisis prompts a request for residential placement or an emergency-room visit. Unfortunately, there are waiting lists and increasing government cutbacks for residential programs across the United States, and a recent review identified fewer than 135 beds in 9 specialized inpatient treatment programs across the country.[16] Yet other programs across the United States and Canada are beginning to demonstrate how to build integrated networks at the regional and state level, which increase expertise and overall system capacity while closing the gap between research and practice.[48] The research reviewed here, combined with more systematic training and more coordinated services, has exciting potential to help limit the impact, if not prevent the emergence, of severe problem behavior.

REFERENCES

1. Baghdadli A, Pascal C, Grisi S, et al. Risk factors for self-injurious behaviours among 222 young children with autistic disorders. J Intellect Disabil Res 2003; 47(8):622–7.
2. Dominick KC, Davis NO, Lainhart J, et al. Atypical behaviors in children with autism and children with a history of language impairment. Res Dev Disabil 2007;28(2):145–62.
3. McTiernan A, Leader G, Healy O, et al. Analysis of risk factors and early predictors of challenging behavior for children with autism spectrum disorder. Res Autism Spectr Disord 2011;5(3):1215–22.
4. Murphy O, Healy O, Leader G. Risk factors for challenging behaviors among 157 children with autism spectrum disorder in Ireland. Res Autism Spectr Disord 2009;3(2):474–82.
5. Richards C, Oliver C, Nelson L, et al. Self-injurious behaviour in individuals with autism spectrum disorder and intellectual disability. J Intellect Disabil Res 2012;56(5):476–89.

6. McClintock K, Hall S, Oliver C. Risk markers associated with challenging behaviours in people with intellectual disabilities: a meta-analytic study. J Intellect Disabil Res 2003;47(6):405–16.

7. Richman DM, Barnard-Brak L, Bosch A, et al. Predictors of self-injurious behaviour exhibited by individuals with autism spectrum disorder. J Intellect Disabil Res 2012;57(5):429–39.

8. Matson JL, Sipes M, Fodstad JC, et al. Issues in the management of challenging behaviours of adults with autism spectrum disorder. CNS Drugs 2011;25(7): 597–606.

9. Emerson E, Kiernan C, Alborz A, et al. Predicting the persistence of severe self-injurious behavior. Res Dev Disabil 2001;22(1):67–75.

10. Hyman SL, Fisher W, Mercugliano M, et al. Children with self-injurious behavior. Pediatrics 1990;85(3):437–41.

11. Kahng S, Iwata BA, Lewin AB. Behavioral treatment of self-injury, 1964 to 2000. Am J Ment Retard 2002;107(3):212–21.

12. Lee LC, Harrington RA, Chang JJ, et al. Increased risk of injury in children with developmental disabilities. Res Dev Disabil 2008;29(3):247–55.

13. Anderson C, Law JK, Daniels A, et al. Occurrence and family impact of elopement in children with autism spectrum disorders. Pediatrics 2012;130(5): 870–7.

14. Hodgetts S, Nicholas D, Zwaigenbaum L. Home sweet home? Families' experiences with aggression in children with autism spectrum disorders. Focus Autism Other Dev Disabl 2013;28(3):166–74.

15. Kalb LG, Stuart EA, Freedman B, et al. Psychiatric-related emergency department visits among children with an autism spectrum disorder. Pediatr Emerg Care 2012;28(12):1269–76.

16. Siegel M, Doyle K, Chemelski B, et al. Specialized inpatient psychiatry units for children with autism and developmental disorders: a United States survey. J Autism Dev Disord 2012;42(9):1863–9.

17. Pennsylvania Bureau of Autism Services. Pennsylvania Bureau of Autism Services. 4; unwanted outcomes—police contact & urgent hospital care. 8-1-2011. Harrisburg, PA, Pennsylvania Department of Public Welfare. Pennsylvania autism needs assessment: a survey of individuals and families living with autism.

18. Sturmey P, Lott JD, Laud R, et al. Correlates of restraint use in an institutional population: a replication. J Intellect Disabil Res 2005;49(7):501–6.

19. Autism and Developmental Disabilities Monitoring Network Surveillance Year 2008 Principal Investigators; Centers for Disease Control and Prevention. Prevalence of autism spectrum disorders—autism and developmental disabilities monitoring Network, 14 sites, United States, 2008. MMWR Surveill Summ 2012; 61(3):1–19.

20. Siegel M, Beaulieu AA. Psychotropic medications in children with autism spectrum disorders: a systematic review and synthesis for evidence-based practice. J Autism Dev Disord 2012;42(8):1592–605.

21. Wink LK, Erickson CA, McDougle CJ. Pharmacologic treatment of behavioral symptoms associated with autism and other pervasive developmental disorders. Curr Treat Options Neurol 2010;12(6):529–38.

22. Canitano R, Scandurra V. Psychopharmacology in autism: an update. Prog Neuropsychopharmacol Biol Psychiatry 2011;35(1):18–28.

23. Doyle CA, McDougle CJ. Pharmacologic treatments for the behavioral symptoms associated with autism spectrum disorders across the lifespan. Dialogues Clin Neurosci 2012;14(3):263–79.

24. Reichow B. Overview of meta-analyses on early intensive behavioral intervention for young children with autism spectrum disorders. J Autism Dev Disord 2012; 42(4):512–20.
25. Matson JL, LoVullo SV. A review of behavioral treatments for self-injurious behaviors of persons with autism spectrum disorders. Behav Modif 2008;32(1): 61–76.
26. Matson JL, Benavidez DA, Compton LS, et al. Behavioral treatment of autistic persons: a review of research from 1980 to the present. Res Dev Disabil 1996;17(6): 433–65.
27. Lilienfeld SO. Scientifically unsupported and supported interventions for childhood psychopathology: a summary. Pediatrics 2005;115(3):761–4.
28. Myers SM, Johnson CP, American Academy of Pediatrics Council on Children with Disabilities. Management of children with autism spectrum disorders. Pediatrics 2007;120(5):1162–82.
29. Sturmey P. Mental retardation and concurrent psychiatric disorder: assessment and treatment. Curr Opin Psychiatry 2002;15(5):489–95.
30. Hagopian LP, Rooker GW, Jessel J, et al. Initial functional analyses outcomes and modifications in pursuit of differentiation: a summary of 176 inpatient cases. J Appl Behav Anal 2013;46(1):88–100.
31. Hanley GP, Iwata BA, McCord BE. Functional analysis of problem behavior: a review. J Appl Behav Anal 2003;36(2):147–85.
32. Iwata BA, Pace GM, Dorsey MF, et al. The functions of self-injurious behavior: an experimental-epidemiological analysis. J Appl Behav Anal 1994;27(2):215–40.
33. Vollmer TR, Hagopian LP, Bailey JS, et al. The association for behavior analysis international position statement on restraint and seclusion. Behav Anal 2011; 34(1):103–10.
34. Hagopian LP, Caruso-Anderson ME. Integrating behavioral and pharmacological interventions for severe problem behavior displayed by children with neurogenetic and developmental disorders. In: Shapiro BK, Accardo PJ, editors. Neurogenetic syndromes: behavioral issues and their treatment. Baltimore (MD): Paul H Brookes Publishing; 2010. p. 217–39.
35. Kurtz PF, Boelter EW, Jarmolowicz DP, et al. An analysis of functional communication training as an empirically supported treatment for problem behavior displayed by individuals with intellectual disabilities. Res Dev Disabil 2011;32(6): 2935–42.
36. Cox A, Brock M, Odom S, et al. National Professional Development Center on ASD: an emerging national educational strategy. In: Doehring P, editor. Autism services across America: road maps for improving state and national education, research, and training programs. Baltimore (MD): Paul H. Brookes Publishing; 2013. p. 249–68.
37. Powers MD, Palmieri MJ, D'Eramo KS, et al. Evidence-based treatment of behavioral excesses and deficits for individuals with autism spectrum disorders. In: Reichow B, Doehring P, Cicchetti DV, et al, editors. Evidence-based practices and treatments for children with autism. New York: Springer Science + Business Media; 2011. p. 55–92.
38. National Autism Center. The national standards project: addressing the need for evidence based practice guidelines for autism spectrum disorders. Randolph (MA): National Autism Center; 2009.
39. Reichow B, Volkmar F, Cicchetti D. Development of the evaluative method for evaluating and determining evidence-based practices in autism. J Autism Dev Disord 2008;38(7):1311–9.

40. Scahill L, McCracken J, McDougle CJ, et al. Methodological issues in designing a multisite trial of risperidone in children and adolescents with autism. J Child Adolesc Psychopharmacol 2001;11(4):377–88.

41. Volkmar FR, Reichow B, Doehring P. Evidence-based practices in autism: where we are now and where we need to go. In: Reichow B, Doehring P, Cicchetti DV, et al, editors. Evidence-based practices and treatments for children with autism. New York: Springer Science + Business Media; 2011. p. 365–91.

42. Doehring P, Winterling V. Delaware autism program: statewide educational services in the public schools. In: Doehring P, editor. Autism services across America: road maps for improving state and national education, research, and training programs. Baltimore (MD): Paul H. Brookes Publishing; 2013. p. 161–84.

43. Reichow B, Doehring P, Cicchetti DV, et al. Evidence-based practices and treatments for children with autism. 2011. xvi, 408 pp.: 2011, p -408.

44. Hagopian LP, Rooker GW, Rolider NU. Identifying empirically supported treatments for pica in individuals with intellectual disabilities. Res Dev Disabil 2011; 32(6):2114–20.

45. Harvey ST, Boer D, Meyer LH, et al. Updating a meta-analysis of intervention research with challenging behaviour: treatment validity and standards of practice. J Intellect Dev Disabil 2009;34(1):67–80.

46. Devlin S, Healy O, Leader G, et al. Comparison of behavioral intervention and sensory-integration therapy in the treatment of challenging behavior. J Autism Dev Disord 2011;41(10):1303–20.

47. Devlin S, Leader G, Healy O. Comparison of behavioral intervention and sensory-integration therapy in the treatment of self-injurious behavior. Res Autism Spectr Disord 2009;3(1):223–31.

48. Doehring P. Autism services across America: road maps for improving state and national education, research, and training programs. Baltimore (MD): Paul H. Brookes Publishing; 2013.

Using Communication to Reduce Challenging Behaviors in Individuals with Autism Spectrum Disorders and Intellectual Disability

Tiffany L. Hutchins, PhD[a],*, Patricia A. Prelock, PhD, CCC-SLP[b,c]

KEYWORDS

- Autism Spectrum Disorder • Intellectual Disability • Communication • Behavior
- Intervention

KEY POINTS

- Individuals with Autism Spectrum Disorder/Intellectual Disability (ASD/ID) are at risk for challenging behaviors that can result from an inability to satisfy their needs through effective communication.
- Communicative impairments in ASD/ID are related to joint attention and the theory of mind difficulties and characterized by profound pragmatic deficits, poor expressive language, and a paucity of communication initiations.
- Evidence-based interventions, such as Functional Communication Training, Interpretive Strategies, the Picture Exchange Communication System and Augmentative and Alternative Communication, and Pivotal Response Training, can support increased communication and decrease challenging behavior.
- It is concluded that an effective communication system will address one or more of the communication deficits of ASD/ID, must be personalized and conducted using a genuine attitude of respect for the individual, and should be effective immediately upon its introduction even if the ultimate goal is to progress to a more sophisticated symbolic system.

Funding Sources: Nil.

Conflict of Interest: Nil.

[a] Department of Communication Sciences and Disorders, University of Vermont, 407 Pomeroy Hall, 489 Main Street, Burlington, VT 05405, USA; [b] Department of Communication Sciences and Disorders, College of Nursing & Health Sciences, University of Vermont, Dean's Office, 105 Rowell Building, 106 Carrigan Drive, Burlington, VT 05405, USA; [c] Pediatrics, College of Medicine, University of Vermont, 105 Rowell Building, 106 Carrigan Drive, Burlington, VT 05405, USA

* Corresponding author.

E-mail address: Tiffany.Hutchins@uvm.edu

INTRODUCTION

Challenging behaviors are a frequent concern for individuals with Autism Spectrum Disorder (ASD) who may or may not have a concomitant intellectual disability (ID). Common challenging behaviors that occur across the lifespan include self-stimulation and stereotypy, self-injury, noncompliance, physical aggression, and other destructive or disruptive behaviors.[1,2] Without appropriate intervention, challenging behaviors tend to persist in individuals with ASD/ID and related developmental disabilities,[2,3] leading to exclusion from education-based and community-based services (and social participation more generally) which, in turn, serves to further limit opportunities for learning and development.[2,4,5] As such, the presence of challenging behaviors has clear implications for treatment planning and the training of parents and professionals who provide services to individuals with ASD/ID.

Crucially, individuals with ASD/ID may use challenging behaviors as a form of expressive communication,[6–8] which is reinforced by the finding that individuals with ASD/ID with higher language skills tend to evidence less frequent and less severe behavioral challenges and interventions that focus on establishing effective communication strategies show reductions in a variety of disruptive behaviors.[9,10] The purpose of this article is to describe the importance of engaging the individual with ASD/ID in a process of communicative development for addressing challenging behaviors. This process is necessary so that the individual "may come to experience, firsthand, the power of communication as an effective tool for satisfying needs and expressing thoughts and feelings."[11(p208)] To support effective communication, and ultimately promote more adaptive behaviors, it is instructive to review the communicative challenges characteristic of ASD/ID first that are relevant for the present purposes.

COMMUNICATION CHALLENGES IN ASD/ID

One difficulty in describing communicative challenges in ASD involves the individual differences in cognitive and linguistic abilities. Some individuals evidence severe cognitive impairments and extremely limited receptive language abilities and are functionally nonverbal. Others outperform neurotypical individuals on verbal and nonverbal tests of intelligence and have precocious vocabularies. Even when language form and content seem to be intact, however, individuals with ASD/ID experience considerable difficulty understanding and using language to express themselves appropriately for the purposes of social communication. Thus, deficits in the pragmatic domain are particularly emblematic of the disorder.[11]

The pragmatic deficits characteristic of autism are partly explained by deficits in receptive language. It is noteworthy that neurotypical children evidence stronger receptive relative to expressive language skills and this pattern has been observed from the earliest stages of development,[12] which makes sense because "language comprehension must always occur ahead of production, as children cannot functionally use words which they do not understand."[13(p682)] Therefore, evidence that receptive skills are impaired relative to expressive skills in ASD[13–15] has important implications for those working to improve adaptive functioning. First, it follows that expressive language strengths can be recruited to improve communication (as in the teaching of appropriate verbal output). Perhaps more importantly, however, it suggests that comprehension can be promoted to scaffold expressive language further while addressing a foundational aspect of language impairment.[13]

Of course, expressive language deficits also occur in ASD/ID particularly in the area of initiation. Although conversational initiation is clearly deficient, not all aspects of initiation are. For example, "a child who hits others or leaves an activity to indicate that he or she wants to be finished with it is initiating even though the behavior is undesirable."[11(p214)] The implication is that effective strategies for using communication to remediate challenging behaviors must provide a way for the individual to initiate communicative exchanges in conventional, or at least transparent, ways.[11]

The pragmatic deficits of ASD/ID are primarily rooted in the developmental events that precede language acquisition and which constitute the basis of pragmatic communication ability. These developmental events include deficits in joint attention[16] and "theory of mind"[17] as well as an inability to integrate and derive meaning from diverse pieces of information in context.[18] That is, typically developing children engage in episodes of joint attention whereby they share attention to an object while monitoring their interactional partner's affect and engagement.[19] They develop a "theory of mind" so as to understand others' mental states, attitudes, and intentional stances. Not only do they instinctively read social cues encoded in the paralinguistic features of language (eg, tone of voice, intonation, and stress patterns), interpret facial expressions and nonverbal gestures, and make inferences about the inner mental worlds of others, but they also relate these cues to the physical and social environment to extract meaningful information and acquire social and cultural knowledge. As discussed more fully later in this article, compensatory strategies to support the sociocultural learning that is acquired by typically developing children through episodes of language-mediated and context-bound joint interactions can be potent for addressing challenging behaviors.

Before leaving the topic of communicative impairments in ASD/ID, it is important to note that communication deficits are related to more general challenges in the ability to process transient stimuli, shift attention, and filter irrelevant information. Accordingly, many popular intervention strategies to support communication and behavior make use of visual supports, capitalizing on this area of relative strength for persons with ASD/ID. Visual supports have been used in a range of contexts to facilitate a variety of communicative interactions, build vocabulary, and help the individual organize his or her thinking. Indeed, visual supports have the potential to lessen cognitive load and enhance understanding and research has demonstrated reductions in challenging behaviors when visual elements are incorporated into treatment plans.[20]

EPIDEMIOLOGY OF CHALLENGING BEHAVIOR IN ASD/ID

"Challenging behaviors" is a term used to describe a heterogeneous set of problem behaviors that vary in their nature, frequency, and severity. Some have characterized challenging behaviors as more demanding or less demanding[21] to reflect this variation but most researchers refer to a relatively uniform set of behaviors that are included under this term. As noted previously, these are self-stimulation and stereotypy, self-injury, noncompliance, physical aggression, and other destructive or disruptive behaviors.

Recent prevalence estimates of challenging behaviors in individuals with ASD/ID range from 35.8% to 64.3% with most studies reporting that more than half of these individuals engage in more than one challenging behavior.[4,5,22,23] Not surprisingly, the severity of challenging behaviors is related to both ASD[24] and ID severity[4,25] and the rates for individuals with ASD and ASD/ID are substantially higher than individuals diagnosed with ID alone (ie, 10%–15%).[21]

USING COMMUNICATION TO ADDRESS BEHAVIORAL CHALLENGES

Several strategies for using communication to remediate the core deficits of ASD/ID have been developed. This article reviews the 4 following intervention categories:

1. Functional communication training (FCT)

2. Interpretive strategies
3. The picture exchange communication system (PECS) and augmentative and alternative communication (AAC)
4. Pivotal response training (PRT)

These approaches differ in their procedures and theoretical focus (and sometimes the targeted population) and, although not all were developed specifically for the purpose of addressing challenging behaviors, all have received an impressive degree of empiric support for this purpose.

Functional Communication Training

At its most basic level, communication is an active effort to affect one's environment. It is "the power to make adaptations and/or bring about change in the human condition."[11(p207)] Carr and Durand[6] were the first to document predictable relationships between environmental circumstances and challenging behaviors. They showed that low levels of adult attention and high levels of task difficulty were associated with misbehavior and that when children were taught to solicit attention and assistance verbally through FCT, problem behaviors were suppressed. The results of this study confirmed the idea that many behavior problems can be viewed as a nonverbal means of communication and that problem behaviors may serve a variety of functions. FCT is designed for anyone who displays challenging behaviors. Nonverbal individuals or those with limited language are taught to communicate using AAC strategies. In this approach, the child's expressive language skills are recruited and the child is trained to initiate communication using carefully selected communicative phrases (or signs or AAC) to replace problem behaviors that presumably serve the same function.

To understand the functions behind a challenging behavior, researchers and service-providers often conduct a Functional Behavior Analysis (FBA). FBA grew out of work in Applied Behavior Analysis and is a process to determine the relationship between events in a person's environment and the occurrence of a challenging behavior so as to develop appropriate intervention strategies.[26,27] Although a variety of functions have been identified in the literature, these are typically collapsed into 1 of 4 primary functions that sometimes go by slightly different names. One scheme uses the terms *Attention* (the goal is to receive attention from others), *Objects and Activities* (the goal is to gain access to a desired object or activity), *Escape/Avoid* (the goal is to escape or avoid something that is perceived as aversive), and *Automatic Reinforcement* (a behavior occurs because it feels good, alleviates pain, or is otherwise internally reinforcing).[8] A variety of FBA procedures have been developed to assess behavioral functions including interviews with persons who are familiar with the child, record review, child observation, and more structured functional analyses.[28] Behavior checklists are completed during some period of observation to examine antecedent events, behavioral responses, and environmental consequences (eg, the Antecedent-Behavior-Consequence checklist,[29] the Motivation Assessment Scale).[30] Generally speaking, FBA has proven to be a valuable tool in the development of treatment plans to address challenging behaviors and research has demonstrated that the use of FBA is associated with improved treatment outcomes.[31]

Interpretive Strategies

People communicate primarily for the purposes of joint attention; to bring another person's focus of attention in alignment with one's own for the purpose of sharing an experience. As noted previously, a deficit in communicating for joint attention is a hallmark impairment of ASD[32] that restricts access to social information and cultural learning. Misperception of social events leads to anxiety, which, in turn, may manifest as "aggressive or oppositional behavior...tantrums, rage, and 'meltdowns'."[33(p123)] Thus, Interpretive Strategies that facilitate communication to give individuals with ASD/ID access to relevant social information are theoretically potent for addressing challenging behaviors.

A variety of Interpretive Strategies have been developed that vary in the nature and degree of structure they provide and the extent to which they invite or require active participation. Interpretive Strategies are adult-mediated activities that make use of visual supports (eg, photos, icons, words, stick drawings, worksheets) to structure a conversation. They can be used after an unsuccessful behavior or situation or before an anticipated challenging situation. Interpretive Strategies are not punishments; they are supportive and constructive and they use a patient and positive tone.[33,34] The purpose of Interpretive Strategies is to help the individual with ASD/ID understand social situations and develop problem-solving skills by reviewing behavioral and social issues using a structured visual format.

Well-liked Interpretive Strategies include (but are by no means limited to) Social Skills Autopsies,[35] the Situation, Options, Consequences, Choices, Strategies, Simulation (SOCCSS),[36] and a subcategory of interventions known as story-based interventions. The most popular story-based interventions are Social Stories[37] and Comic Strip Conversations.[38] Each strategy is summarized in **Table 1**.

The PECS and AAC Strategies

PECS[39] is an aided picture/icon-based augmentative system designed to teach communicative initiations for a variety of communicative functions (eg, requesting objects, answering questions, commenting). PECS is designed for individuals who are nonverbal or who have the limited language abilities to "address fundamental and pivotal communication problems, namely, the failure to initiate communication."[40(p258)] By contrast, the more general class of AAC strategies should be considered for anyone with ASD/ID[41] to support expression and comprehension. Of course, given the tremendous individual differences in ASD/ID, AAC interventions should always be tailored to the individual's communicative needs.[42]

Table 1	
Interpretive strategies for supporting social communication	
Interpretive Strategy	**Description**
Social autopsies[35]	Following a social mistake, the individual completes a worksheet with an adult to identify the mistake, determine who was harmed and how to correct the mistake, and develop a plan to prevent the mistake in the future.
SOCCSS[36]	Following a social problem, the individual completes a worksheet with an adult to identify the situation (ie, who, what, when, where, and why), brainstorm alternative behavior options, identify the consequences of each, prioritize these options, develop a plan to carry out the option, and practice the behavior.
Story-based intervention[37,38]	Personalized stories are constructed for or with the individual to give the individual direct access to social information with the idea that advances in social cognition should be accompanied by more appropriate behaviors. Story-based interventions need not focus on problem behaviors and affirmative stories that celebrate social success and offer praise are encouraged.

A few popular AAC strategies take the form of simple visual supports that communicate choices, expectations for behaviors, or directives. These strategies are known to most practitioners and include things like contingency maps (essentially if/then statements), scripts (eg, "How to brush my teeth"), and the First/Then strategy. These strategies may be effective in managing behavior because they make use of simple and readily understood visuals to communicate basic information. On the other hand, they are not designed to support or encourage reciprocal communication and initiation, which does not mean that these strategies are undesirable last resorts. To the contrary, there are simply situations whereby these pragmatic options need to be available. It does mean that these strategies occupy a lower rung on the symbolic hierarchy. Although this may make them advantageous for certain individuals or situations, they must be used in the context of a more comprehensive approach that aims to build a communication system in which the individual can *initiate* communication in adaptive ways.

PRT

Communication requires a degree of motivation that individuals with ASD/ID often lack. PRT[43] focuses on increasing motivation by incorporating child choice, turn-taking, and direct and natural reinforcers that are directly related to the task. Maintenance tasks are also interspersed with novel tasks to ensure the individual experiences success and enjoyment during communicative exchanges. Originally designed to promote language development through the use of behavioral principles, the idea is to target pivotal behaviors such as motivation and communication initiations that lead to large collateral changes in untargeted areas of functioning. Individuals who respond well to PRT tend to have an interest in toys and low to moderate levels of nonverbal stereotypy and moderate to high rates of verbal stereotypy.[44]

CLINICAL VIGNETTE: COMMUNICATION STRATEGIES TO ADDRESS CHALLENGING BEHAVIORS

When we met 8-year-old "Kevin" (pseudonym), he had been diagnosed with autism and had low-average language skills according to formal testing. Our intervention with Kevin focused on the challenging behavior of pinching. As a first step in developing the intervention, we engaged in an information-gathering process that included child observation and an in-depth interview with Kevin's mother. We also engaged Kevin in a series of Comic Strip Conversations[39] to explore the causes and consequences of the pinching behavior from his perspective.

Through maternal interview, child observation, and our own structured conversations with Kevin, we learned a great deal about the purposes behind and contexts surrounding his pinching behavior. Kevin pinched family members and children and adults at school when he was excited, bored, anxious, or angry. As such, pinching seemed to fall into the category of Automatic Reinforcer with the behavior related to sensory sensitivities and self-dysregulation. Pinching was a daily occurrence and, although Kevin had been told on several occasions that pinching was not acceptable, the pinching had persisted and increased in frequency. Kevin was aware and saddened by the fact that his pinching was often painful to others but reported that he was simply unable to stop.

Based on the information gathered, we developed a Social Story[34,37] to communicate to Kevin what was happening during these pinching events. Care was taken to ensure that the language level was appropriate and that the words chosen would be meaningful and accurate. Visual supports in the form of BoardMaker symbols were added to take advantage of the visual processing strengths characteristic of ASD. Kevin's Social Story is presented in the Appendix to this article.

Data for a 4-week baseline (A) and 6-week Social Story intervention phase (B) are presented in Fig. 1. Subjective data in the form of behavior ratings and maternal daily diaries were

collected across AB phases of study. Kevin's mother was asked to rate Kevin's ability to resist pinching across settings on a scale of 1 to 10 (higher values indicating more positive outcomes).

Data from this pre-experimental design reveal that maternal subjective ratings of positive behaviors increased from 4.0 during baseline to 8.2 during intervention with many days with no pinching during intervention. Several of the mother's reports support the rating data and suggest qualitative shifts in Kevin's understanding of, and ability to engage in discussions about, pinching. For example, one report read, "No pinching all day. He began to ask questions about when he first started pinching. We talked about other behaviors that he used to have (biting, scratching, pushing) that he's learned not to do. Kevin agrees that the [social] story is very true to what he does and how he feels." Other comments during this period revealed how Kevin was using strategies provided in the Social Story, including, "He did not pinch me today. Instead he buried his face into my chest and began to squeeze me. He wanted to pinch me during homework this evening…but he snapped instead (on his own, no prompt!)."

Intervention using Social Stories was immediately effective and although pinching was not totally eliminated during intervention (see **Fig. 1**), Kevin's mother was nevertheless enthusiastic about the therapeutic changes she had seen in Kevin's behavior and understanding. This is exemplified in her comment that, "If you would have told me a year ago that we would be able to go a full day without pinching I would have said that was crazy. We have many days now of no pinching at all!"

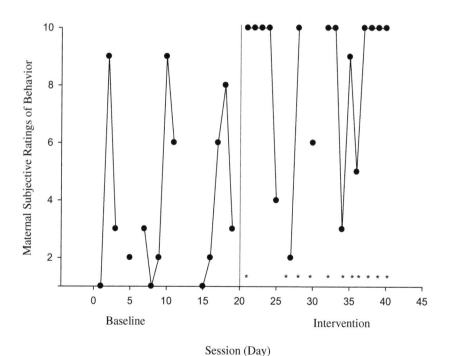

Fig. 1. Maternal subjective ratings of pinching behavior for A (baseline) and B (intervention) phases using a 10-point scale with higher values indicating less problematic behavior. Asterisks indicate the days on which the Social Story was read.

This example highlights some important considerations for using communication to address challenging behaviors. First, it illustrates the use of an Interpretive Strategy for creating meaning-making in socially and culturally relevant ways. Second, it underscores the importance of the information-gathering process and the assemblage of meaningful and accurate information.[34] Third, this example illustrates the importance of adopting an attitude of genuine respect for the individual; one that recognizes the unique perspective of the individual and uses this as a framework to developing a personalized treatment plan.[11] Finally, Kevin's story reminds us of the power of communication and social learning for facilitating introspection and analysis to support more optimal outcomes. Indeed, this mother's reports (and similar reports from parents reported elsewhere[45,46]) support the notion that Interpretive Strategies like Social Stories and Comic Strip Conversations can assist the individual in thinking through challenging situations and problem behaviors to help them make more adaptive behavioral decisions.

REVIEW OF CURRENT EVIDENCE

The interventions described in this article were selected by their strong empiric support. All of the interventions (with a few exceptions noted below for specific treatment strategies within the broader intervention class) have been identified by the National Standards Project[47] as established treatments for ASD. Established treatments are those for which a high level of evidence is available and abundant. In short, they are interventions for which several well-controlled studies have been shown to produce beneficial effects, although, to our knowledge, only Social Stories[48] and PECS[49] have been the subject of randomized controlled trials.

FCT

There are nearly 200 studies, including several reviews, with evidence to support positive outcomes for individuals with ASD/ID and related disorders when using FCT to address challenging behavior.[50–54] FCT meets the criteria for being considered a well-established treatment across a range of challenging behaviors.[51,53,55–58] There are some potential unwanted effects, however, when using FCT. Namely, overuse of the newly trained response or return of the unwanted behavior is possible if reinforcement is delayed or insufficient to meet the original communicative need.[50]

Interpretive Strategies

With regard to Interpretive Strategies, Social Skills Autopsies[35] and SOCCSS[36] have not been evaluated adequately with reports of their effectiveness coming mainly from practitioners.[33] As noted above, Social Stories have been rigorously evaluated and story-based interventions have been identified as 1 of 11 established treatments in ASD/ID by the National Standards Project.[47] They have been found to be effective for addressing a wide range of problem behaviors in school and home settings,[3,46] including disruptive behaviors,[59] tantrums,[46] aggression,[60] and self-injurious acts.[61] It should be noted that tremendous variability in effect size within and across studies has been observed with scant evidence with regard to which participant characteristics predict success.[63,64] Some evidence is accumulating, however, that the concreteness of the target and the clarity with which stories can be written is one predictor of success.[31,62] Although originally intended for individuals with high functioning ASD,[37] more recent evidence confirms that Social Stories and Comic Strip Conversations can be used successfully for individuals who are nonverbal and have the most severe challenges.[60,62,64]

PECS and AAC

Research investigating both PECs and AAC demonstrates effectiveness in supporting the communication of children with ASD who have limited or no functional communication. Much of the efficacy research for PECS reports positive outcomes for increasing verbalizations and social initiations as well as decreasing problem behaviors.[65–69] Researchers have investigated the impact of PECS on the ability to exchange pictures, use words spontaneously,[70,71] make requests,[72,73] and decrease inappropriate behaviors.[69] Not all results, however, are consistently observed for all study participants, highlighting the importance of recognizing and addressing individual variation and needs.

The use of AAC with individuals with ASD has a growing body of evidence,[74] although it is often not immediately considered for individuals with ASD/ID because of fears that speech development will be hindered.[41,75] Millar and coworkers[76] reported, however, that AAC is an effective strategy for decreasing challenging behavior without limiting the development of speech in individuals with ASD and related disorders.

PRT

PRT has strong evidence for supporting parent education and facilitating social communication. Children with ASD have been taught to imitate words that, generalized across settings,[77] improve their speech intelligibility,[78] decrease their tantrums and physical aggression,[20,78,79] and increase their social communication.[80,81]

DISCUSSION

In a vital sense, there is no distinction between communication and behavior. The act of communication itself is behavioral and all observed behaviors, whether they are intended as communicative, have message value. Herein lies a major challenge (and source of anxiety) for individuals with ASD/ID who lack recognition, not only of this relationship between communication and behavior,[82] but also of the power of communicative behaviors for shared meaning-making, cultural learning, and satisfying needs more generally.

This article considered several strategies for using communication to address challenging behaviors in ASD/ID. Each approach targeted one or more of the communication impairments characteristic of ASD/ID, which contribute to deficits in the pragmatic domain. Whichever strategy is used, the authors agree with Twatchman[11] that a genuine attitude of respect for the individual and his/her perspective must be adopted. There are misunderstandings between people and what is called challenging behaviors that makes perfect sense when viewed by the person with autism. In short, an attitude of respect and nonjudgment helps toward understanding the reasons behind maladaptive behaviors so that they may be addressed effectively and with the most careful consideration.

With the exception of a few AAC strategies, all of the reviewed approaches are designed to support communication initiation; this is critically important because initiation provides a means for affecting one's environment and satisfying needs. As described previously, communication strategies—even those that do not support reciprocity and initiation—can be effective for some purposes; however, the authors strongly suggest that they be viewed as one tool in a larger communication system that supports the ability to initiate communication in more conventional ways. At the same time, the communication system should be effective at reducing challenging behaviors from the moment of its introduction even if the ultimate goal is to progress to a more sophisticated symbolic system,[11] which also does not mean that a focus on the foundational processes of joint attention and shared meaning-making cannot be emphasized. In fact, strategies like joint attention training can be beneficial for all individuals with ASD/ID and may be particularly important for those with the most limited language skills.[83] Of course, creating opportunities for joint attention and promoting a child's functional language understanding is likely to be a more challenging and less immediately rewarding task for the interventionist. Nevertheless, "such an approach will focus on addressing the child's fundamental, rather than the more outwardly observable, aspects of a language impairment."[13(p688)]

SUMMARY AND FUTURE DIRECTIONS

The literature is promising in the area of communication intervention to address challenging behaviors in individuals with ASD/ID. The interventions described in this article are evidence-based and highly feasible for addressing behavioral challenges across settings. The empiric research, however, usually involves children, with little investigation of adult populations—a much-needed area of research foci. In a related vein, interventions with individuals with ASD/ID are not uniformly effective. Thus, an important direction for research involves identifying the participant, context, and intervention variables that predict success with communicative strategies to address challenging behaviors. It will also be important to continue the investigation of interventions that specifically address the challenging behaviors that are common in individuals with ASD/ID while capturing the critical role that communication or the lack of communication plays.

REFERENCES

1. Fodstad JC, Rojahn J, Matson JL. The emergence of challenging behavior in at-risk toddlers with and without autism spectrum disorder: a cross sectional study. J Dev Phys Disabil 2012;24:217–34.
2. Horner RG, Carr EG, Strain PS, et al. Problem behavior interventions for young children with autism: a research synthesis. J Autism Dev Disord 2002;32: 423–46.
3. Machalicek W, O'Reilly MF, Beretvas N, et al. A review of interventions to reduce challenging behavior in school settings for students with autism spectrum disorders. Res Autism Spectr Disord 2007;1:229–49.
4. Holden B, Gitlesen JP. A total population study of challenging behavior in the count of Hedmark, Norway: prevalence and risk markers. Res Dev Disabil 2006;27:456–65.
5. Murphy O, Healy O, Leader G. Risk factors for challenging behaviors among 157 children with autism spectrum disorder in Ireland. Res Autism Spectr Disord 2009;3:474–82.
6. Carr EG, Durand VM. Reducing behavior problems through functional communication training. J Appl Behav Anal 1985;18:111–26.
7. Chaing H. Expressive communication of children with autism: the use of challenging behavior. J Intellect Disabil Res 2008;52:966–72.
8. Glasberg BA. Stop that seemingly senseless behavior: FBA-based interventions for people with autism. Bethesda (MD): Woodbine House; 2008.
9. Koegel LK, Koegel R. The child with autism as an active communication partner: child-initiated strategies for improving communication and reducing behavior problems. In: Koegel LK, Koegel R, editors. Psychosocial treatments for child

and adolescent disorders: empirically based strategies for clinical practice. Washington, DC: American Psychological Association; 1996. p. 553–72.

10. Koegel LK, Koegel RL, Surratt A. Language intervention and disruptive behavior in preschool children with autism. J Autism Dev Disord 1992;22:141–53.

11. Twatchman JL. Improving the human condition through communication training in autism. In: Cautela JR, Ishaq BW, editors. Contemporary issues in behavior therapy: improving the human condition. New York: Plenum Press; 1996. p. 207–31.

12. Fenson L, Dale PS, Reznick JS, et al. Variability in early communicative development. Monogr Soc Res Child Dev 1994;59:1–185.

13. Hudry K, Leadbitter K, Temple K, et al. Research report: preschoolers with autism show greater impairment in receptive compared to expressive language abilities. Int J Lang Commun Disord 2010;45:681–90.

14. Charman T, Drew A, Baird C, et al. Measuring early language development in preschool children with autism spectrum disorder using the MacArthur Communicative Development Inventory. J Child Lang 2003;30:213–36.

15. Luyster RJ, Kadlec MB, Carter A, et al. Language assessment and development in toddlers with autism spectrum disorders. J Autism Dev Disord 2008;38: 1426–38.

16. Jones EA, Carr EG. Joint attention in children with autism: theory and intervention. Focus Autism Other Dev Disabl 2004;19:13–26.

17. Miller C. Developmental relationships between language and theory of mind. Am J Speech Lang Pathol 2006;15:142–54.

18. Brock J, Norbury C, Einav S, et al. Do individuals with autism process words in context? Evidence from language-mediated eye-movements. Cognition 2008; 108:896–904.

19. Tomasello M. Constructing a language. Cambridge (MA): Harvard University Press; 2003.

20. Dettmer S, Simpson R, Myles B, et al. The use of visual supports to facilitate transitions of students with autism. Focus Autism Other Dev Disabl 2000;15:163–9.

21. Emerson E, Kiernon C, Alborz A, et al. The prevalence of challenging behaviors: a total population study. Res Dev Disabil 2001;22:77–93.

22. Baghdadli A, Pascal PS, Aussillous GC. Risk factors for self-injurious behaviors among 222 young children with autistic disorders. J Intellect Disabil Res 2009; 47:622–7.

23. Lecavalier L. Behavioral and emotional problems in young people with pervasive developmental disorders: relative prevalence, effects of subject characteristics, and empirical classification. J Autism Dev Disord 2006;36:1101–14.

24. Bodfish JW, Symons FJ, Parker DE, et al. Varieties of repetitive behavior in autism: comparisons to mental retardation. J Autism Dev Disord 2000;30:237–43.

25. Borthwick-Duffy SA. Prevalence of destructive behaviors. In: Thompson T, Gray DB, editors. Destructive behavior in developmental disabilities: diagnosis and treatment. Thousand Oaks (CA): Sage; 1994. p. 2–23.

26. O'Neill RE, Horner RH, Albin RW, et al. Functional behavioral analysis of problem behavior: a practical assessment guide. Pacific Grove (CA): Brookes/Cole; 1990.

27. Rogers E. Functional behavioral assessment and children with autism: working as a team. Focus Autism Other Dev Disabl 2001;16:228–31.

28. Buschbacher PW, Fox L. Understanding and intervening with the challenging behavior of young children with autism spectrum disorder. Lang Speech Hear Serv Sch 2003;34:217–27.

29. Miltenberger RG. Behavior modification: principles and procedures. Pacific Grove (CA): Brookes/Cole; 1997.

30. Durand VM, Crimmins DB. The motivation assessment scale. Topeka (KS): Monaco & Associates; 1992.

31. Kokina A, Kern L. Social Story™ interventions for students with autism spectrum disorders. J Autism Dev Disord 2010;40:812–26.

32. Wetherby AM, Prizant BM, Schuler AL. Understanding the nature of communication and language impairments. In: Wetherby AM, Prizant BM, editors. Autism spectrum disorders: a transactional developmental perspective. Baltimore (MD): Paul H. Brookes; 2005. p. 109–42.

33. Myles B. Behavioral forms of stress management for individuals with Asperger syndrome. Child Adolesc Psychiatr Clin N Am 2003;12:123–41.

34. Gray C. The new social story™ book. Arlington (TX): Future Horizons; 2010.

35. Lavoie R. Social skill autopsies: a strategy to promote and develop social competencies. Available at: http://www.ldonline.org/article/14910/2005. Accessed December, 2012.

36. Roosa JB. Men on the move: competence and cooperation. Conflict resolution and beyond. Author: Kansas City (MO); 1995.

37. Gray C, Garand JD. Social stories: improving responses of students with autism with accurate social information. Focus Autistic Behav 1993;8:1–10.

38. Gray C. Comic strip conversations. Arlington (TX): Future Horizons; 1994.

39. Bondy A, Frost L. The picture exchange communication system. Focus Autistic Behav 1994;9:1–19.

40. Simpson RL, Ganz JB. Picture exchange communication system (PECS). In: Prelock PA, McCauley RJ, editors. Treatment of autism spectrum disorders: evidence-based intervention strategies for communication and social interaction. Baltimore (MD): Paul H. Brookes; 2012. p. 255–80.

41. Wegner JR. Augmentative and alternative communication strategies: manual signs, picture communication, and speech-generating devices. In: Prelock PA, McCauley RJ, editors. Treatment of autism spectrum disorders: evidence-based intervention strategies for communication and social interaction. Baltimore (MD): Paul H. Brookes; 2012. p. 27–48.

42. Mirenda P. Introduction to AAC for individuals with autism spectrum disorders. In: Mirenda P, Iacono T, editors. Autism spectrum disorders and AAC. Baltimore (MD): Paul H. Brookes; 2009. p. 3–22.

43. Koegel RL, Koegel LK. Pivotal response treatments for autism: communication, social, and academic development. Baltimore (MD): Paul H. Brookes; 2006.

44. Sherer M, Schreibman L. Individual behavior profiles and predictors of treatment effectiveness for children with autism. J Consult Clin Psychol 2005;73:525–38.

45. Hutchins TL, Prelock PA. Using social stories and comic strip conversations to promote socially valid outcomes for children with autism. Semin Speech Lang 2006;27:47–59.

46. Hutchins TL, Prelock PA. Supporting theory of mind development: considerations and recommendations for professionals providing services to individuals with autism spectrum disorder. Top Lang Disord 2008;28:340–64.

47. National Autism Center. National standards project – findings and conclusions: addressing the needs for evidence-based practice guidelines for autism spectrum disorder. Randolph (MA): National Autism Center; 2009. Available at: http://www.naiotnalautismcenter.org. Accessed December, 2012.

48. Quirmbach LM, Lincoln AJ, Feinberg-Gizzo MJ, et al. Social stories: mechanisms of effectiveness in increasing game play skills in children diagnosed with autism spectrum disorders using a pretest posttest repeated measures randomized control group design. J Autism Dev Disord 2009;39:299–321.

49. Howlin P, Gordon RK, Pasco G, et al. The effectiveness of Picture Exchange Communication System (PECS) training for teachers of children with autism: a pragmatic, group randomized controlled trial. J Child Psychol Psychiatry 2007;48:473–81.

50. Durand VM. Functional communication training: treating challenging behavior. In: Prelock PA, McCauley RJ, editors. Treatment of autism spectrum disorders: evidence-based intervention strategies for communication and social interaction. Baltimore (MD): Paul H. Brookes; 2012. p. 107–38.

51. Matson JL, Dixon DR, Matson ML. Assessing and treating aggression in children and adolescents with developmental disabilities: a 20-year overview. Educ Psychol 2005;25:151–81.

52. Mirenda P. Supporting individuals with challenging behavior through functional communication training and AAC: research review. Augment Altern Commun 1997;13:207–25.

53. Petscher ES, Rey C, Bailey JS. A review of empirical support for differential reinforcement of alternative behavior. Res Dev Disabil 2009;30:409–25.

54. Smith T, Scahill L, Dawson G, et al. Designing research studies on psychosocial interventions in autism. J Autism Dev Disord 2007;37:354–66.

55. Durand VM, Merges E. Functional communication training to treat challenging behavior. In: O'Donohue W, Fisher JE, editors. Cognitive behavior therapy: applying empirically supported techniques in your practice. New York: John Wiley & Sons; 2008. p. 222–9.

56. Durand VM, Merges E. Functional communication training to treat challenging behavior. In: O'Donohue W, Fisher JE, editors. General principles and empirically supported techniques of cognitive behavior therapy. New York: John Wiley & Sons; 2009. p. 320–7.

57. Halle JW, Ostrosky MM, Hemmeter ML. Functional communication training: a strategy for ameliorating challenging behavior. In: McCauley RJ, Fey ME, editors. Treatment of language disorders in children. Baltimore (MD): Paul H. Brookes; 2006. p. 509–48.

58. Mancil GR. Functional communication training: a review of the literature related to children with autism. Educ Train Dev Disabil 2006;41:213–24.

59. Scattone D, Wilczynski SM, Edwards RP, et al. Decreasing disruptive behaviors of children with autism using social stories. J Autism Dev Disord 2002;32:535–43.

60. Swaggart BL, Gagnon E, Bock SJ, et al. Using social stories to teach social ad behavioral skills to children with autism. Focus Autistic Behav 1995;10:1–15.

61. Del Valle PR, McEachern AG, Chambers HD. Using social stories with autistic children. J Poetry Ther 2001;14:187–97.

62. Hutchins TL, Prelock PA. The social validity of Social Stories™ for supporting the behavioural and communicative functioning of children with autism spectrum disorder. Int J Speech Lang Pathol 2013;15(4):383–95.

63. Reynhout G, Carter M. Evaluation of the efficacy of Social Stories™ using three single subject metrics. Res Autism Spectr Disord 2011;5:885–900.

64. Barry LM, Burlew SB. Using social stories to teach choice and play skills to children with autism. Focus Autism Other Dev Disabl 2004;19:45–51.

65. Beck AR, Stoner JB, Bock SJ, et al. Comparison of PECS and the use of a VOCA: a replication. Educ Train Dev Disabil 2008;43:198–216.

66. Carr D, Felce J. Brief report: the effects of PECS teaching to phase III on the communicative interactions between children with autism and their teachers. J Autism Dev Disord 2007;37:724–37.

67. Carr D, Felce J. Brief report: increase in production of spoken words in some children with autism after PECS teaching to phase III. J Autism Dev Disord 2007;37:780–7.
68. Charlop-Christy MH, Carpenter M, Le L, et al. Using the Picture Exchange Communication System (PECS) with children with autism: assessment of PECS acquisition, speech, social-communicative behavior, and problem behavior. J Appl Behav Anal 2002;35:213–31.
69. Ganz JB, Simpson RL. Effects on communication requesting and speech development of the picture exchange communication system in children with characteristics of autism. J Autism Dev Disord 2004;34:395–408.
70. Yoder P, Stone WL. A randomized comparison of the effect of two prelinguistic communication interventions on the acquisition of spoken communication in preschoolers with ASD. J Speech Lang Hear Res 2006;49:698–711.
71. Tincani M. Comparing the Picture Exchange Communication System and sign language training for children with autism. Focus Autism Other Dev Disabl 2004;19:152–63.
72. Yoder P, Stone WL. Randomized comparison of two communication interventions for preschoolers with autism spectrum disorders. J Consult Clin Psychol 2006;74:426–35.
73. Mirenda P, Iacono T. Autism spectrum disorders and AAC. Baltimore (MD): Paul H. Brookes Publishing Co; 2009.
74. Millar DC, Light JC, Schlosser RW. The impact of augmentative and alternative communication intervention on the speech production of individuals with developmental disabilities: a research review. J Speech Lang Hear Res 2006;49: 248–69.
75. Millar D. Effects of AAC on the natural speech development of individuals with autism spectrum disorders. In: Mirenda P, Iacono T, editors. Autism spectrum disorders and AAC. Baltimore (MD): Paul H. Brookes Publishing Co; 2009. p. 171–92.
76. Koegel RL, Dyer K, Bell L. The influence of child-preferred activities on autistic children's social behavior. J Appl Behav Anal 1987;20:243–52.
77. Koegel RL, Camarata S, Koegel LK, et al. Increasing speech intelligibility in children with autism. J Autism Dev Disord 1998;28:241–51.
78. Koegel LK, Koegel R, Hurley C, et al. Improving social skills and disruptive behavior in children with autism through self-management. J Appl Behav Anal 1992;25:341–53.
79. Oke N, Schreibman L. Training social initiations to a high-functioning autistic child: assessment of collateral behavior change and generalization in a case study. J Autism Dev Disord 1990;20:479–97.
80. Bruinsma Y. Increases in the joint attention behavior of eye gaze alternation to share enjoyment as a collateral effect of pivotal response treatment for three children with autism [Unpublished doctoral dissertation]. Santa Barbara (CA): University of California; 2004.
81. Stahmer A. Teaching symbolic play skills to children with autism using pivotal response training. J Autism Dev Disord 1995;25:123–41.
82. Twatchman-Cullen D. Communication and stress in students with autism spectrum disorders. In: Baron M, Groden J, Groden G, et al, editors. Stress and coping in autism. New York: Oxford University Press; 2006. p. 302–22.
83. Twatchman-Cullen D, Twatchman-Reilly J. Communication and language issues in less able school-age children with autism. In: Gabriels RL, Hill DE, editors. Growing up with autism. New York: Guilford Press; 2007. p. 73–94.

APPENDIX

Kevin's Social Story

What to do when I want to pinch?

My name is Kevin.

I am 9 years old and I go to [name of school].

I know lots of people at home and at school.

Sometimes when I am at home or school or somewhere else, I might pinch someone.

Sometimes I pinch because it makes me feel relaxed, like when I snuggle with my Mom.

Sometimes I pinch when I get excited, like when I goof around with [stepsister] and [dog's name] or wrestle with [stepfather].

Other times, I pinch when I am bored and tired of waiting.

When I pinch, this can make others think, "Hmmm, that's strange." "I wasn't expecting that." "I wonder why Kevin pinched me."

They might also think, "Ouch! That hurts!" or "I wish he wouldn't do that."

I have worked hard with [interventionist] to learn how to stop pinching.

When I want to pinch at home, I can talk to my mom about it.

I can also hug my mom or squeeze her hand.

I might also do a thumb-war or a hand massage to help me stop pinching.

When I want to pinch at school, I can snap my fingers.

I can also tell [school SLP's name] that I feel like pinching and she can try to help me to stop.

I am still learning how not to pinch and that is ok.

It makes my Mom happy when I do things that help me stop pinching.

Examination of Aggression and Self-injury in Children with Autism Spectrum Disorders and Serious Behavioral Problems

Devon Carroll, MSN[a], Victoria Hallett, PhD[b],
Christopher J. McDougle, MD[c], Michael G. Aman, PhD[d],
James T. McCracken, MD[e], Elaine Tierney, MD[f],
L. Eugene Arnold, MD, MEd[d], Denis G. Sukhodolsky, PhD[g],
Luc Lecavalier, PhD[d], Benjamin L. Handen, PhD, BCBA-D[h],
Naomi Swiezy, PhD[i], Cynthia Johnson, PhD[h], Karen Bearss, PhD[j],
Benedetto Vitiello, MD[k], Lawrence Scahill, MSN, PhD[j],*

KEYWORDS

- Aggression • Self-injury • Autism • Disruptive behavior

Statistical Analysis: Victoria Hallett, PhD; Lawrence Scahill, MSN, PhD.

This work was funded by National Institute of Mental Health by the following RUPP grants: Yale, U10MH66764; Indiana University, U10MH66766; Ohio State University, U10MH66768. Johnson & Johnson Pharmaceutical Research & Development provided active risperidone for the study. This publication was also supported by the Yale CTSA, UL1 RR024139; IU CTSA, UL1 RR025761; OSU CTSA, UL1 RR025755 from the National Center for Research Resources.

Disclaimer: The opinions and assertions contained in this article are the private views of the authors and are not to be construed as official or as reflecting the views of the Department of Health and Human Services, the National Institutes of Health, or the National Institute of Mental Health.

Disclosures: Dr Scahill, Roche, consultant; Bracket, consultant, BioMarin, consultant; speaker's honoraria from the Tourette Syndrome Association; Roche, research support; Pfizer, research support; research support and study drug supply from Shire. Dr Aman, Roche, consultant; Bristol-Meyers Squibb, consultant, research grant; Forest, consultant; Pfizer, consultant; Supernus, consultant; Johnson & Johnson, research grant. Dr McDougle, study drug supply from Shire. Dr McCracken, research support from Seaside Therapeutics, Roche, and Otsuka; consultant income from Novartis, BioMarin, PharmaNet, and Noven; speaker's honoraria from the Tourette Syndrome Association; research support and study drug supply from Shire. Dr Arnold, AstraZeneca, advisory board; Biomarin, advisory board; CureMark, research funding; Forest, research funding; Lilly, research funding; Noven, advisory board; Seaside therapeutics, advisory board; Shire, research funding. Dr Tierney, BioMarin, consultant. Dr Handen has received research support from Eli Lilly, Curemark, and Bristol-Myers Squibb. Drs Hallett, Lecavalier, Sukhodolsky, Bearss, Johnson, Swiezy, and Vitiello report no financial relationships with commercial interests.

[a] Family & Children's Aid, Danbury, CT, USA; [b] Kings College in London, London, UK; [c] Harvard University, MA, USA; [d] Ohio State University, OH, USA; [e] University of California at Los Angeles, CA, USA; [f] Kennedy-Krieger in Baltimore, MD, USA; [g] Yale University, CT, USA; [h] University of Pittsburgh, PA, USA; [i] Indiana University, IN, USA; [j] Emory University, GA, USA; [k] National Institute of Mental Health, MD, USA

* Corresponding author. Marcus Center, 1920 Briarcliff Road, Atlanta, GA 30329.
E-mail address: lawrence.scahill@emory.edu

KEY POINTS

- Aggression and self-injurious behavior (SIB) are common in children with autism spectrum disorder (ASD) and impair adaptive function.
- Typologies such as proactive (cold) aggression and reactive (hot) aggression have been described, but not previously applied to ASD.
- This study identified subtypes of aggression in a sample of 206 children with ASD (aged 5–17 years) who participated in 2 risperidone trials conducted by the Research Units on Pediatric Psychopharmacology Autism Network.
- Five subtypes emerged: hot aggression only, cold aggression only, SIB only, aggression and SIB, and nonaggression. However, these groups are not mutually exclusive because children may show aggression or SIB in different categories.
- Despite some differences in clinical characteristics across subtypes, all groups showed a positive response to risperidone.

INTRODUCTION

Pervasive developmental disorders (PDDs) are lifelong neurodevelopmental conditions characterized by impairments in social interaction and communication skills, as well as repetitive behavior and unusual preoccupations.[1] In Diagnostic and Statistical Manual of Mental Disorders, Fifth Edition (DSM-V), the former diagnostic classifications of autistic disorder, PDD–not otherwise specified (PDD-NOS) and Asperger disorder will be collapsed into a single category called autism spectrum disorder (ASD), reflecting their common features and potentially shared causes. Recent estimates of prevalence indicate that ASDs affect as many as 110 per 10,000 children.[2]

In addition to the core symptoms, children with ASDs may have other problems including tantrums, aggression, self-injury, hyperactivity, anxiety, or rapid changes in mood.[3] The prevalence of aggressive behavior in this population varies widely depending on the source of sample and method of assessment.[4–8] Whether directed toward the self or others, aggression may result in injury and distress for the child and caregivers. Aggression is a common chief complaint of parents and educators.[9] Behavioral treatment of aggression can be challenging, expensive, and often requires expertise that may not be available in all communities.[10] Although 2 atypical antipsychotic medications, risperidone and aripiprazole, are approved by the US Food and Drug Administration (FDA) for the treatment of irritability (tantrums, aggression, and self-injury), these medications are associated with short-term and long-term adverse effects.[5,11–13] In addition, medication withdrawal of risperidone after 6 months of effective treatment resulted in the rapid return of disruptive behaviors.[14]

Pharmacologic studies on the treatment of aggression generally do not discriminate between types of aggressive behaviors.[12,15,16] The randomized, controlled risperidone and aripiprazole trials that led to FDA approval enrolled children with autistic disorder with any combination of tantrums, aggression, and self-injury as measured by the Aberrant Behavior Checklist (ABC) Irritability subscale.[12,17–19] Although the term irritability implies an affective component, these studies did not evaluate the context of the tantrums, aggression, and self-injury. In contrast, behaviorists are focused on the context or the function of the behavior.[20] For example, the function of an aggressive outburst may be to obtain a tangible object (food or a preferred object) or to escape an environmental demand (getting dressed). Self-injury (aggression directed at the self) occurs in some children with ASDs and may occur with or without externally directed aggression. Functional analysis is also relevant to self-injurious behavior (SIB).[20–22] The repetitive motoric nature of SIB in some children suggests that it may differ from other types of aggressive behavior.[20]

In behavioral science, research has focused on subtypes of aggression in order to understand the underlying mechanisms.[23] The classic taxonomy originating from animal research distinguishes between predatory (proactive) and affective (reactive) aggression. The characteristics of reactive and proactive aggression have been studied in animal models and in humans.[23–25] Proactive aggression (cold aggression) is intended to achieve a desired reward and, in its classic form, occurs without anger or prior provocation.[23,26,27] Reactive, or hot-headed aggression, occurs in response to a perceived or real provocation and is often impulsive.[23–25] However, these subtypes of aggression may not be mutually exclusive.[23,28] In ASD, for example, the child who is intent on obtaining a preferred object, may over-react and become aggressive in the effort to obtain the object.

The reactive and proactive subtypes of aggression have been studied in the general pediatric population and, to a lesser extent, in clinical samples.[29,30] To date, most studies of aggression in clinical samples have focused on children with attention-deficit/hyperactivity disorder, oppositional defiant disorder, and conduct disorder.[25,31,32] Research on aggression subtypes in children with ASDs is limited.[7,8] In a sample of 1380 children with ASD aged 4 to 17 years from the Simons Simplex data base, Kanne and Mazurek[7] estimated the prevalence of current aggression at 35%. This estimate was based on a single item from the Autism Diagnostic Interview–Revised. Parents were asked to rate aggression on a 4-point scale (0, none; 1, mild; 2, moderate; 3, severe). The 35% estimate reflects the percentage of children rated 2 or 3 on this item. A secondary analysis of the Autism Treatment Network data (N = 1584; ages 2–17 years) estimated a prevalence of aggression of 53.7% based on a yes or no response from parents on a single question about aggression. This higher rate likely includes children with mild aggression, who were not counted in the estimate of 35% from the Simons Simplex data base. These reports did not attempt to classify the types of aggression or SIB in these samples of children with ASD.

In this analysis we examine aggressive behavior in children who participated in the 2 risperidone trials conducted by the Research Units on Pediatric Psychopharmacology (RUPP) Autism Network.[12,15]

First, we classified subtypes of aggression and self-injury based on the parents' chief complaint documented at baseline. Second, we examined differences in these subtypes by comparing demographic and clinical characteristics by subtype. Third, we explored treatment response to risperidone across subgroups.

METHODS
Setting and Subjects

Subjects were enrolled in 1 of 2 randomized clinical trials conducted by the RUPP Autism Network. The first study was an 8-week, double-blind, placebo-controlled trial of risperidone in 101 children 5 to 17 years old with autistic disorder. The second study was a 24-week randomized trial of risperidone only versus risperidone plus parent training in 124 children with ASDs from 4 to 13 years of age. Medication dosing and blinded assessments in these two studies were virtually identical for the first 8 weeks, which permitted comparison of baseline characteristics and outcomes across the two trials. Both studies required the presence of serious behavioral problems such as tantrums, aggression, or self-injury in various combinations, as shown by a score of 18 or higher on the Aberrant Behavior Checklist–Irritability subscale (ABC-I). This score is approximately 1.3 standard deviation units more than the population mean for individuals with developmental disabilities.[33,34]

The two trials included a total of 225 subjects (187 boys, 38 girls). Subjects in both studies were free of serious medical disorders or other psychiatric disorders requiring medication. All children were drug free for 7 to 28 days, depending on the drug (7 days for stimulants and alpha 2 agonists, 28 days for fluoxetine or antipsychotics), before randomization. Thus, with the exceptions of including subjects with broader ASD diagnosis and narrower age range in the second trial, the two studies had similar entry criteria. The design of each trial, the risperidone dosing schedule, and the characteristics of the samples are described in detail in prior reports.[12,15,35,36] Both projects were approved by institutional review boards at participating clinical sites. Parents or legal guardians of all child participants provided written informed consent.

Measures

Before randomization, participants in both trials received a comprehensive psychiatric and medical evaluation (including electrocardiogram, vital signs, medical history, physical examination, and routine laboratory tests). Diagnoses of autistic disorder, Asperger disorder, and PDD-NOS were based on a clinical evaluation according to Diagnostic and Statistical Manual of Mental Disorders, Fourth Edition (DSM-IV)[37] or DSM-IV–Text Revision (DSM-IV-TR)[1] criteria. The diagnoses were further supported by the Autism Diagnostic Interview–Revised (ADI-R).[38] The following assessment battery was used to confirm eligibility, characterize the sample, and establish baseline severity.

Parent target problems

At baseline, the clinician asks parents to identify 1 or 2 chief complaints concerning their children's behavior. Parents are then asked to describe the frequency, duration (or time spent), intensity and impact of the behavior on daily function or family life. This description was documented in a brief narrative at baseline, which was used as baseline for an outcome measure of change over time.[39] However, for classifying aggression and SIB in this study, we used only the baseline narratives from these two trials.

Intellectual functioning

Based on the child's capacity to complete the test, several different intelligence tests were used including Stanford Binet-V,[40] Wechsler Intelligence Scales for Children–III,[41] Leiter International Performance Scale–Revised,[42] Mullen Scales of Early Learning,[43] Slosson Intelligence Test,[44] and Wechsler Preschool and Primary Scale of Intelligence–Revised.[45] Because several different tests were used, children were classified into 2 intelligence quotient (IQ) categories: less than 70 or greater than or equal to 70.

Clinical Global Impressions scale

The Clinical Global Impressions (CGI)–Severity (CGI-S) scale is a clinician-rated 7-point measure of overall severity, ranging from 0 (normal) to 7 (extreme).[46] A score of 4, reflecting moderate or greater disturbance, was required for study inclusion. The CGI-Improvement (CGI-I) scale is a clinician-rated scale designed to assess change from baseline, based on all available sources of information. Scores range from very much improved (1) through no change (4) to very much worse (7). In keeping with convention, a score of much improved or very much improved was used to define positive response.

Autism Diagnostic Interview-Revised
The Autism Diagnostic Interview–Revised (ADI-R) is a reliable and valid structured parent interview used to support the diagnosis of autistic disorder.[38,47,48] The interview inquires about reciprocal social interaction, communication, restricted interests, and repetitive behavior. In these RUPP Autism Network trials, interviews were administered and scored by clinicians trained to reliability.

Vineland Adaptive Behavior Scales
The Vineland is a semistructured parent interview designed to assess functioning in 3 domains: communication, daily living skills, and socialization. This instrument is a standard assessment tool and has shown excellent reliability and validity.[49]

ABC
The ABC is a 58-item rating scale that is completed by a parent or teacher. The ABC has normative data in children with developmental disabilities[33] and is sensitive to change in this population.[12,15] Items are rated on a 4-point scale ranging from 0 (not a problem) to 3 (the problem is severe). There are 5 factor-analyzed subscales: Irritability (15 items), Social Withdrawal (16 items), Stereotypic Behavior (7 items), Hyperactivity (16 items), and Inappropriate Speech (4 items). The Irritability subscale surveys aggression, self-injury, tantrums, and unstable mood. Scores range from 0 to 45; high scores indicate high levels of symptom severity.[34]

Children's Yale-Brown Obsessive-Compulsive Scale for PDDs
The Children's Yale-Brown Obsessive-Compulsive Scale (CYBOCS) is a semistructured, clinician-rated interview designed to assess the current severity of obsessions and compulsions in youth with obsessive-compulsive disorder.[50] In the risperidone trials, the CYBOCS was modified for use in children with ASDs.[51] The modified CYBOCS does not include the checklist or severity scales for obsessions, but retains the checklist and severity scales for compulsions. The 5 severity items include time spent, interference, distress, resistance, and degree of control, each rated from 0 to 4. This scale yields a single total score from 0 to 20.[51]

Procedures

Classification of parent target problems
Coding proceeded in several steps. First, 2 coders (DC, LS) examined 20 parent target problems (PTPs) from 10 randomly selected cases. By consensus, these raters proposed 6 categories and then independently classified all available baseline PTPs into 1 of these 6 categories. Disagreements were resolved by consensus.

Given that each subject had 2 PTPs, a subject could have 0, 1, or 2 problems with aggression or SIB. To create mutually exclusive groups, children were classified as follows: (1) hot aggression only (1 PTP indicated hot aggression, the other did not involve aggression or SIB), (2) cold aggression only (1 PTP indicated cold aggression, the other did not involve aggression, SIB, or tantrums), (3) SIB only, (4) hot and cold aggression (1 PTP reflected hot aggression, the other reflected cold aggression), (5) aggression and SIB (1 PTP reflected aggression, the other reflected self-injury), (6) nonaggression (neither PTP reflected aggression or SIB; eg, tantrums not involving aggression or SIB). **Table 1** presents examples of PTPs at baseline and their classification in this study. These classifications were based on inferences by the study coders (DC, LS). Parents were not directly asked to comment on the classification of hot or cold aggression.

Table 1
Selected examples of PTPs for participants in RUPP Autism Network risperidone trials

Problem	Description	Impact/Consequences	Classification
Tantrums	Occur at home and school. Behaviors include swearing, destruction of toys, slamming doors, and throwing things. May hit mother or sibling	Occur 10–15 times per day; lasting 5 to 20 min. Parents may have to restrain him to calm him down	Hot aggression
Impulsive aggression	Includes pulling at mother's glasses, pulling hair, and hitting (mother or sister). Behavior is unpredictable	Occurs daily up to 5 times per day. Mother tells him "No" and sends him to the time-out chair	Cold aggression
Self-injury	Scratches and bites himself about 3 times per day. Gets upset when he does not get his way, or when sitting in time-out. Hits his head against the wall	Daily: makes holes in the walls; leaves marks or draws blood	SIB (hot subtype)
Screaming and outbursts	Has outbursts every day at least once an hour. Has a screaming outburst if he wants something, if he wants someone to leave him alone, and for no apparent reason at times. Only stops if something distracts him	Episodes last seconds to 10 min. Family can only go to places where screaming is acceptable (eg, Magic Mountain). Behavior interferes with learning	Nonaggression
Impulsiveness	Near constant. Mother says: "Hundreds of episodes per day." Behavior is dangerous, because he may dart into the road or bolt in parking lots	Wearing on the family, hard to do the simplest errands with the child, family avoids taking the child to outings such as grocery store	Nonaggression

Abbreviation: RUPP, Research Units on Pediatric Psychopharmacology.

Analytical Strategy

Demographic characteristics (age, gender, race and ethnicity, and educational placement) and clinical characteristics (ASD diagnosis; IQ category <70 or ≥70; scores on the CGI-S, Vineland, ADI-R, ABC, and CYBOCS-PDD; heart rate and blood pressure) were evaluated in the available sample.

Inter-rater agreement for the independent coding of the individual PTPs (2 per child) was evaluated with Cohen's kappa, which corrects for chance.[52] Once the frequency of PTP categories was established, subtypes were compared on demographic and clinical characteristics. Continuous variables were evaluated by analysis of covariance (ANCOVA) (controlling for IQ) across aggression subtypes. Pair-wise differences were investigated using Tukey's post hoc comparisons, and χ^2 tests were used for categorical variables. A repeated measures mixed model was used to determine the main effects of group (aggression subtype) and time (baseline and week 8) and the group-time interaction on the ABC Irritability subscale in risperidone-treated subjects (ie, subjects on placebo in the first RUPP trial were not included in the analysis). To assess treatment response by aggression subtype on the CGI-I (positive response = score of much improved or very much improved) at week 8, we conducted a series of pair-wise comparisons. The hot aggression, cold aggression, SIB, and aggression plus SIB were each compared with the nonaggression group. These analyses also did not include subjects assigned to placebo in the first trial.

RESULTS
Sample Characteristics

Because of missing or incomplete PTPs for 19 subjects at baseline, the present analyses included 206 children (174 boys, 32 girls). **Table 2** presents demographic and clinical characteristics for this sample.

Inter-rater agreement on the classification of aggression subtypes was good (kappa, 0.77; 95% confidence interval [CI], 0.71, 0.84]). **Table 3** presents the frequency of the aggression subtypes: hot aggression only (n = 65), cold aggression only (n = 32), SIB only (n = 33), aggression plus SIB (n = 17), nonaggression (n = 53). Children with reported hot and cold aggression were excluded (n = 6) from **Table 3** and all subsequent analyses owing to the small number and difficulty of placing them in either group.

There were no significant differences on gender ($\chi^2_{(4)}$ = 2.60, P = .63), ethnicity ($\chi^2_{(16)}$ = 18.23, P = .31) or ASD diagnosis ($\chi^2_{(8)}$ = 11.82, P = .16) across the 5 groups (the 6 subjects with hot and cold aggression were not included). There were also no group differences in the available physiologic measures of heart rate ($F_{(4,188)}$ = 0.80; P = .53) and systolic blood pressure ($F_{(4,179)}$ = 0.34; P = .85).

The χ^2 analysis showed group differences by IQ ($\chi^2_{(4)}$ = 10.06, $P<.05$). Pair-wise comparisons showed that the aggression plus SIB group had a higher proportion of children with IQs less than 70 (82%) compared with the following groups: hot aggression only (48%; $\chi^2_{(1)}$ = 6.41; P = .01), cold aggression only (47%; $\chi^2_{(1)}$ = 6.30; P = .01), and nonaggression (5%; $\chi^2_{(4)}$ = 8.11; $P<.01$). Children with reported SIB only were also more likely to have an IQ less than 70 (67%) compared with the nonaggression group (47%; $\chi^2_{(4)}$ = 3.75; P = .05). Age differed significantly across aggression types ($F_{(4,199)}$ = 2.42; P = .05). This finding was driven by the marginally younger group with hot aggression (mean 7.29 ± 2.27 years) compared with the nonaggression group (mean 8.61 ± 2.49 years; P = .06). No other pair-wise comparisons were significant on post hoc testing.

With adjustment for IQ, the omnibus ANCOVA was significant on the ABC Irritability subscale ($F_{(4,180)}$ = 5.11; $P<.01$). Pair-wise comparisons by subtype confirmed that children in the aggression plus SIB group had significantly higher ABC irritability scores (mean 33.00 ± 7.91) than children in the nonaggression group (mean 25.50 ± 7.00; $P<.05$). The general pattern suggests that the children with aggression plus SIB are more severely affected (see **Table 3**). However, after adjusting for IQ, other ABC subscales, Vineland scores, CYBOCS-PDD scores, CASI PDD, and anxiety scores were not different across groups.

The rate of positive response to risperidone (CGI-I rating of much improved or very much improved) was not significantly different across the 5 groups ($\chi^2_{(4)}$ = 1.45; P = .84). **Table 4** shows the rate of positive and negative response to risperidone by aggression subtype. As shown in **Table 4**, the positive response to risperidone was high in all groups and there were no significant differences between groups with aggressive behavior, SIB, or the combination compared with the nonaggression group.

Fig. 1 shows the change in ABC Irritability in each of the aggression subtypes in the risperidone treatment groups. The mean scores in the placebo group are also

Table 2
Demographic and clinical characteristics of all participants in RUPP risperidone trials

	Mean	SD
Age (y)	7.98	2.70
	N	**%**
Gender		
Male	174	84.5
Female	32	15.5
Race and Ethnicity		
White	149	72.3
Black	16	7.8
Hispanic	25	12.1
Asian/Pacific Islander	9	4.4
Other	7	3.4
Educational Placement		
Regular education	47	22.8
Regular education, some special education services	72	35.0
Special education school	62	30.1
Home school	9	4.4
No school	14	6.8
IQ[a]		
<70	110	53.4
≥70	84	40.8
ASD Diagnosis		
Autistic disorder	163	79.1
Asperger disorder	8	3.9
PDD-NOS	35	17.0
CGI-S		
4 (moderate)	51	24.8
5 (marked)	99	48.1
6 (severe)	54	26.2
7 (extreme)	2	1.0
	Mean	**SD**
ABC[b]		
Irritability	27.82	7.16
Social withdrawal	16.36	8.69
Stereotypy	9.22	5.15
Hyperactivity	34.29	8.88
Inappropriate speech	5.93	3.75
Vineland		
Communication	51.93	20.29
Daily living skills	43.19	19.79
Socialization	53.48	15.21

(continued on next page)

Table 2 (continued)		
CYBOCS-PDD		
Total score	15.22	3.16
CASI		
PDD	23.04	7.14
Anxiety	15.40	9.58

There were missing data on baseline target problem in 19 subjects.
Abbreviation: SD, standard deviation.
[a] Missing IQ data for 12 subjects.
[b] Higher scores indicate greater behavioral problems.

shown for comparison. In the risperidone-treated groups, there was a significant effect of time (baseline vs week 8: $F_{(1,221)} = 144.59$; $P<.01$) and aggression group ($F_{(4,221)} = 3.14$; $P<.05$). The aggression group–time interaction was not significant ($F_{(4,221)} = 0.39$; $P>.05$).

DISCUSSION

This study was designed to identify subtypes of aggression in a sample of children with ASD who participated in 2 multisite trials of risperidone funded by the National Institute of Mental Health (NIMH) conducted by the RUPP Autism Network.[12,15] The classification of aggression subtypes was based on a semistructured narrative derived from parent-reported chief complaint at baseline in each study. Five subtypes of aggression emerged: hot aggression only, cold aggression only, SIB only, aggression and SIB, and nonaggression. Approximately 3% of the sample were classified with both hot and cold aggression and were dropped from the analysis. The most common subtype of aggression in this sample selected for moderate or greater levels of irritability was hot aggression. Children in the hot aggression group had higher scores on ABC Irritability subscale than those without a chief complaint of aggression. Children with aggression and SIB had the highest ABC Irritability subscale scores. Children with IQs less than 70 were more likely to show SIB, either alone or in combination with aggression. The hot aggression group was significantly, albeit slightly, younger than the nonaggression group. The percentage rate of positive response to risperidone was not different across groups as measured by a rating of much improved or very much improved on the CGI-I. All risperidone-treated groups showed improvement on the ABC Irritability subscale with no differences across groups. Given the selection criteria and the large treatment effects of risperidone in these trials, the finding of no group differences in clinical response is not surprising.

Our classification of hot aggression, which occurred in the context of tantrums, is conceptually similar to reactive aggression in youth without developmental disabilities.[26,28,53] Cold aggression in this ASD population, which seems to be driven by interest in a preferred object or escape from routine demand without a report of explosive behavior, could be analogous to proactive aggression.[26,28,53] However, cold aggression in this sample was a default classification in some cases (ie, occurring without a report of explosive behavior), which may have resulted in some misclassification. Proactive aggression is also associated with predatory aggression (premeditated acts of coercion, attacks with purpose to steal, or bullying).[28,54] The degree to which acts of cold aggression are predatory, premeditated, or antisocial in children

Table 3
Demographic and clinical characteristics of 200[a] children with ASDs

	Characteristic	Hot Aggression Only		Cold Aggression Only		Self-injury Only		Self-injury and Aggression		Nonaggression		χ^2	P Value
		n	%	n	%	n	%	n	%	n	%		
Gender	Male	55	84.6	25	78.1	26	78.8	15	88.2	47	88.7	2.60	.63
	Female	10	15.4	7	21.9	7	21.2	2	11.8	6	11.3		
IQ[b]	<70	31	47.7	15	46.9	22	66.7	14	82.4	24	45.3	10.94	.03[c]
	≥70	28	43.1	15	46.9	10	30.3	2	11.8	27	50.9		
ASD diagnosis	Autistic disorder	54	83.1	23	71.9	27	81.8	16	94.1	37	69.8	11.82	.16
	Asperger disorder	2	3.1	0	0	1	3.0	0	0	5	9.4		
	PDD-NOS	9	13.8	9	28.1	5	15.2	1	5.9	11	20.8		

	Characteristic	Hot Aggression Only		Cold Aggression Only		Self-injury Only		Self-injury and Aggression		Nonaggression		F Value[d]	P Value
		Mean	SD	Mean	SD	Mean	SD	Mean	SD	Mean	SD		
Age (y, mo)		7.29	2.27	7.72	2.61	8.11	3.25	8.89	3.39	8.61	2.49	2.42	.05
Vineland	Communication	54.54	20.17	53.16	17.52	47.42	17.81	38.53	15.46	55.66	22.59	1.11	.36
	Daily living skills	45.85	20.58	41.88	15.46	42.45	21.41	33.59	16.61	44.74	21.11	0.87	.48
	Socialization	55.69	13.82	54.47	12.26	52.70	16.39	41.59	16.72	55.68	15.80	1.83	.13
ABC	Irritability	27.98	6.89	27.38	7.94	29.70	5.54	33.00	7.91	25.38	7.01	5.11	<.01[e]
	Social withdrawal	15.25	8.96	15.47	8.43	18.39	8.52	17.35	9.95	16.74	8.52	0.67	.61
	Stereotypy	8.81	5.33	9.59	5.46	8.61	4.64	12.24	4.70	9.11	5.25	1.18	.32
	Hyperactivity	34.76	8.18	34.75	8.51	32.52	9.20	35.41	9.18	34.09	10.10	0.48	.75
	Inappropriate speech	6.33	3.81	5.85	3.61	5.39	3.99	5.18	3.84	6.02	3.65	0.77	.55
CYBOCS-PDD	Total score	15.45	2.96	14.50	2.70	15.21	3.24	14.53	4.24	15.45	3.33	0.73	.57
CASI	Anxiety scale	15.91	10.97	15.45	9.60	15.05	8.82	12.78	7.02	15.83	9.11	0.07	.99
	PDD scale	22.84	6.85	22.81	6.92	22.71	7.30	27.06	5.84	22.37	7.72	0.82	.52
Cardiovascular indices	Heart rate (bpm)	100.20	13.94	102.00	14.81	96.80	14.79	103.35	27.65	96.79	17.55	0.82	.52
	Blood pressure (mm Hg)	107.29	13.88	106.81	13.07	108.04	15.07	105.50	18.52	104.29	11.41	0.34	.85

Abbreviation: bpm, beats per minute.
[a] Six participants with both hot and cold aggression were not included in the analysis.
[b] Missing IQ data for 12 subjects.
[c] P<.05.
[d] ANCOVA analyses controlling for IQ (more than and less than 70). ANCOVA for age did not covary for IQ.

Table 4
Rate of positive and negative response on CGI-I for risperidone-treated subjects in RUPP trials by aggression subtype[a]

Group	Positive Response on CGI-I[b] N (%)	Negative Response on CGI-I[c] N (%)	Chi Square (Compared with Nonaggression Group)	P Value
Nonaggression	33 (58.9)	23 (41.1)	—	—
Hot aggression	45 (69.2)	20 (30.8)	0.63	.43
Cold aggression	22 (68.75)	10 (31.25)	0.37	.54
SIB	20 (60.6)	13 (39.4)	0.02	.88
Any aggression plus any SIB	10 (58.8)	7 (41.2)	0.06	.80

[a] Does not include placebo group.
[b] Positive response = much improved or very much improved on CGI-I.
[c] Negative response = all other CGI-I ratings.

with ASD may be difficult to determine. Thus, cold aggression in ASD may diverge from the traditional construct of proactive aggression. In some children with ASD, cold aggression may be impulsive in nature rather than planned. Moreover, hot and cold aggression may serve similar functions (tangible object or escape from routine demand), but hot aggression reflects the added problem of poor emotion regulation.

The most severely affected group in this sample included children with aggression and SIB. These children were more likely to have intellectual disability, had higher baseline ABC Irritability scores, and lower Vineland communication and Vineland

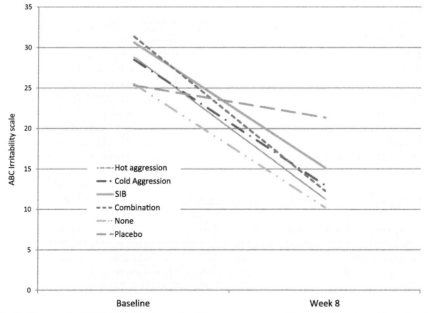

Fig. 1. Change in ABC irritability in each of the aggression subtypes in the risperidone treatment groups (combination = hot aggression + SIB).

socialization scores. It is reassuring that this severely affected group showed a similar rate of positive response to other aggression subgroups. When we defined on a post hoc basis a subgroup of hot aggression and hot SIB, this group also showed a high rate of positive response to risperidone. These results suggest that risperidone is a blunt intervention that exerts positive effects in children with ASD with serious behavioral problems in the context of hot aggression, cold aggression, and tantrums in the absence of aggression. This finding runs counter to clinical lore that medication intervention is more likely to be effective for reactive than proactive aggression. The concept has not been carefully tested (even in a post hoc manner as we have done) and warrants further empirical evaluation.

Limitations

This study offers new information about subtypes of aggression in children with ASDs, but several limitations should be noted. First, these subtypes were constructed after reviewing written descriptions by clinicians following an open-ended inquiry about the child's 2 most important problems. The purpose of documenting the narratives was not focused on classifying subtypes of aggression. If clinicians had been engaged in this endeavor, they may have obtained more, or even different, information. Thus, although the level of agreement on classification of aggression was high, our method of inquiry may have missed information that could have influenced the classification.

Second, this was a convenience sample with known and unknown biases. The study sample included subjects with serious behavioral problems, which threatens the ability to generalize our findings to the wider ASD population. The entry criteria for these two trials required subjects to have increased scores on the ABC Irritability subscale. This criterion may have limited the detection of differences by aggression subgroup. A wider sample of children with ASDs with a broader range of behavioral disturbances is needed to confirm the validity of aggression subtypes in ASD.

Third, the classification strategy used in the current study was intended to create mutually exclusive groups. Although the target problem narratives evaluated here support the existence of aggression subtypes, the narratives only documented 2 problems. Inquiry about a third problem could have identified a problem in another aggressive subtype and affected classification. In typically developing youth and youth with ASD, hot and cold aggression are highly correlated.[28,29] Thus, the placement of subjects in one or another subtype results in some misclassification and makes it difficult to find differences between groups. A dimensional measure of aggression collected in a larger and more diverse population of children with developmental disabilities would be a way to learn more about the subtypes of aggression in children with ASDs.

SUMMARY

The results of this study support, but do not confirm, the subtypes of hot and cold aggression in children with ASDs. These subtypes, which were adapted from previous studies on aggression outside the realm of ASDs, may be useful to guide further study on biological mechanisms and individualized treatment. Overall, our data suggest that aggression subtypes respond similarly to treatment with risperidone. Future studies could examine whether targeting the inadequate emotion regulation of children with hot aggression would lead to benefit from less potent medications or behavioral interventions.[25]

ACKNOWLEDGMENTS

NIMH: Ann Wagner, PhD. Yale: James Dziura, PhD; Lily Katsovich, MS, MBA; Yanhong Deng, MPH; Allison Gavaletz, BA.

REFERENCES

1. American Psychiatric Association. Diagnostic and statistical manual of mental disorders. text revision. 4th edition. Washington, DC: American Psychiatric Association; 2000.
2. Autism and Developmental Disabilities Monitoring Network. Prevalence of autism spectrum disorders—Autism and Developmental Disabilities Monitoring Network, 14 sites, United States, 2012. MMWR Surveill Summ 2012;61(3):1–19. Available at: www.cdc.gov/mmwr/pdf/ss/ss6103.pdf. Accessed February 4, 2013.
3. LeCavalier L. Behavioral and emotional problems in young people with pervasive developmental disorders: relative prevalence, effects of subject characteristics, and empirical classification. J Autism Dev Disord 2006;36: 1101–14.
4. Dominick KC, Davis NO, Lainhart J, et al. Atypical behaviors in children with autism and children with a history of language impairment. Res Dev Disabil 2007;28:145–62.
5. Parikh MS, Kolevzon A, Hollander E. Psychopharmacology of aggression in children and adolescents with autism: a critical review of efficacy and tolerability. J Child Adolesc Psychopharmacol 2008;18:157–78.
6. Hartley SL, Sikora DM, McCoy R. Prevalence and risk factors of maladaptive behaviour in young children with autistic disorder. J Intellect Disabil Res 2008; 52:819–29.
7. Kanne SM, Mazurek MO. Aggression in children and adolescents with ASD: prevalence and risk factors. J Autism Dev Disord 2011;41:926–37.
8. Mazurek MO, Kanne SM, Wodka EL. Physical aggression in children and adolescents with autism spectrum disorders. Res Autism Spectr Disord 2013;7: 455–65.
9. Lecavalier L, Leone S, Wiltz J. The impact of behaviour problems on caregiver stress in young people with autism spectrum disorders. J Intellect Disabil Res 2006;50:172–83.
10. Siegel M, Beaulieu A. Psychotropic medications in children with autism spectrum disorders: a systematic review and synthesis for evidence based practice. J Autism Dev Disord 2012;42:1592–605.
11. Correll CU, Manu P, Olshanskiy V, et al. Cardiometabolic risk of second-generation antipsychotic medications during first-time use in children and adolescents. JAMA 2009;302:1765–73.
12. Research Units on Pediatric Psychopharmacology Autism Network. Risperidone in children with autism and serious behavioral problems. N Engl J Med 2002; 347:314–21.
13. Martin A, Scahill L, Anderson GM, et al. Weight and leptin changes among risperidone-treated youths with autism: 6-month prospective data. Am J Psychiatry 2004;161:1125–7.
14. Research Units on Pediatric Psychopharmacology Autism Network. Risperidone treatment of autistic disorder: longer-term benefits and blinded discontinuation after 6 months. Am J Psychiatry 2005;162:1361–9.

15. Aman MG, McDougle CJ, Scahill L, et al. Medication and parent training in children with pervasive developmental disorders and serious behavior problems: results from a randomized clinical trial. J Am Acad Child Adolesc Psychiatry 2009;48:1143–54.

16. Jensen PS, Youngstrom EA, Steiner H, et al. Consensus report on impulsive aggression as a symptom across diagnostic categories in child psychiatry: implications for medication studies. J Am Acad Child Adolesc Psychiatry 2007;46: 309–22.

17. Marcus RN, Owen R, Kamen L, et al. A placebo-controlled, fixed-dose study of aripiprazole in children and adolescents with irritability associated with autistic disorder. J Am Acad Child Adolesc Psychiatry 2009;48:1110–9.

18. Owen R, Sikich L, Marcus RN, et al. Aripiprazole in the treatment of irritability in children and adolescents with autistic disorder. Pediatrics 2009;124:1533–40.

19. Pandina GJ, Aman MG, Findling RL. Risperidone in the management of disruptive behavior disorders. J Child Adolesc Psychopharmacol 2006;16:379–92.

20. Iwata BA, Dorsey MF, Slifer KJ, et al. Toward a functional analysis of self-injury. J Appl Behav Anal 1994;27:197–209.

21. Schreibman L. Intensive behavioral/psychoeducational treatments for autism: research needs and future directions. J Autism Dev Disord 2000;30:373–8.

22. Machalicek W, O'Reilly MF, Beretvas N, et al. A review of interventions to reduce challenging behavior in school settings for students with autism spectrum disorder. Res Autism Spectr Disord 2007;1:229–46.

23. Krusei MJ, Keller S, Jensen JA. Neurobiology of aggression. In: Martin A, Scahill L, Kratochvil CJ, editors. Pediatric psychopharmacology: principles and practice. 2nd edition. New York: Oxford University Press; 2011. p. 211–25.

24. Moyer KE. Kinds of aggression and their physiological basis. Commun Behav Biol 1968;2:65–87.

25. King S, Waschbusch DA, Pelham WE, et al. Subtypes of aggression in children with attention deficit hyperactivity disorder: medication effects and comparison with typical children. J Clin Child Adolesc Psychol 2009;38:619–29.

26. Dodge KA. The structure and function of reactive and proactive aggression. In: Pepler DJ, Rubin KH, editors. The development and treatment of childhood aggression. Hillsdale (NJ): Lawrence Erlbaum Associates; 1991. p. 201–18.

27. Dodge KA, Lochman JE, Harnish JD, et al. Reactive and proactive aggression in school children and psychiatrically impaired chronically assaultive youth. J Abnorm Psychol 1997;106:37–51.

28. Ollendick TH, Jarrett MA, Wolff JC, et al. Reactive and proactive aggression: cross-informant agreement and the clinical utility of different informants. J Psychopathol Behav Assess 2009;31:51–9.

29. Farmer CA, Aman MG. Aggressive behavior in a sample of children with autism spectrum disorders. Res Autism Spectr Disord 2011;5:317–23.

30. McAuliffe MD, Hubbard JA, Rubin RM, et al. Reactive and proactive aggression: stability of constructs and relations to correlates. J Genet Psychol 2006;167: 365–82.

31. Kempes M, Matthys W, de Vries H, et al. Reactive and proactive aggression in children–a review of theory, findings and the relevance for child and adolescent psychiatry. Eur Child Adolesc Psychiatry 2005;14:11–9.

32. Connor DF, Chartier KG, Preen EC, et al. Impulsive aggression in attention-deficit/hyperactivity disorder: symptom severity, co-morbidity, and attention-deficit/hyperactivity disorder subtype. J Child Adolesc Psychopharmacol 2010;20:119–26.

33. Brown EC, Aman MG, Havercamp SM. Factor analysis and norms for parent ratings on the Aberrant Behavior Checklist-Community for young people in special education. Res Dev Disabil 2002;23:45–60.
34. Aman MG, Singh NN, Stewart AW, et al. Psychometric characteristics of the aberrant behavior checklist. Am J Ment Defic 1985;89:492–502.
35. Scahill L, Aman MG, McDougle CJ, et al. Trial design challenges when combining medication and parent training in children with pervasive developmental disorders. J Autism Dev Disord 2009;39:720–9.
36. Scahill L, McCracken J, McDougle CJ, et al. Methodological issues in designing a multisite trial of risperidone in children and adolescents with autism. J Child Adolesc Psychopharmacol 2001;11:377–88.
37. American Psychiatric Association. Diagnostic and statistical manual of mental disorders. 4th edition. Washington, DC: American Psychiatric Association; 1994.
38. Le Couteur A, Lord C, Rutter M. The autism diagnostic interview-revised (ADI-R). Los Angeles (CA): Western Psychological Services; 2003.
39. Arnold LE, Vitiello B, McDougle C, et al. Parent-defined target symptoms respond to risperidone in RUPP autism study: customer approach to clinical trials. J Am Acad Child Adolesc Psychiatry 2003;42:1443–50.
40. Roid GH. Stanford Binet intelligence scales. 5th edition. Itasca (IL): Riverside Publishing; 2003.
41. Wechsler D. Manual for the Wechsler intelligence scale for children. 3rd edition. San Antonio (TX): Psychological Corporation; 1991.
42. Roid GH, Miller LJ. Leiter international performance scale-revised: examiner's manual. Wood Dale (IL): Stoelting Co; 1997.
43. Mullen E. The Mullen scales of early learning. Circle Pines (MN): American Guidance Service; 1995.
44. Jensen JA, Armstrong RJ. Slosson intelligence test for children and adults. East Aurora (NY): Slosson Educational Publications; 1985.
45. Wechsler D. Manual for the Wechsler preschool and primary scale of intelligence-revised. San Antonio (TX): Psychological Corporation; 1989.
46. Guy W. Clinical global impressions. In: ECDEU Assessment manual for psychopharmacology-revised (DHEW Publ No ADM 76-338). Rockville (MD): US Department of Health, Education, and Welfare, Public Health Service, Alcohol, Drug Abuse, and Mental Health Administration, NIMH Psychopharmacology Research Branch, Division of Extramural Research Programs; 1976. p. 218–22.
47. Lord C, Pickles A, McLennan J, et al. Diagnosing autism: analyses of data from the Autism Diagnostic Interview. J Autism Dev Disord 1997;27:501–17.
48. Research Units on Pediatric Psychopharmacology Autism Network. A randomized, double-blind, placebo-controlled, crossover trial of methylphenidate in children with hyperactivity associated with pervasive developmental disorders. Arch Gen Psychiatry 2005;62:1266–74.
49. Sparrow S, Balla D, Cicchetti D. Vineland Adaptive Behavior Scales. Circle Pines (MN): American Guidance Service; 1984.
50. Scahill L, Riddle MA, McSwiggin-Hardin M, et al. Children's Yale-Brown Obsessive Compulsive Scale: reliability and validity. J Am Acad Child Adolesc Psychiatry 1997;36:844–52.
51. Scahill L, McDougle CJ, Williams SK, et al, Research Units on Pediatric Psychopharmacology Autism Network. Children's Yale-Brown Obsessive Compulsive Scale modified for pervasive developmental disorders. J Am Acad Child Adolesc Psychiatry 2006;45:1114–23.

52. Fleiss JL, Levin B, Paik MC. Statistical methods for rates and proportions. 3rd edition. New York: John Wiley & Sons; 2003.
53. Dodge KA, Coie JD. Social-information-processing factors in reactive and proactive aggression in children's peer groups. J Pers Soc Psychol 1987;53: 1146–58.
54. Vitiello B, Stoff DM. Subtypes of aggression and their relevance to child psychiatry. J Am Acad Child Adolesc Psychiatry 1997;36:307–15.

Psychopharmacologic Management of Serious Behavioral Disturbance in ASD

Kimberly A. Stigler, MD

KEYWORDS

- Autism • Autism spectrum disorders • Aggression • Irritability • Self-injury
- Psychopharmacology

KEY POINTS

- Individuals with autism spectrum disorder (ASD) frequently exhibit serious behavioral disturbance (irritability) involving severe tantrums, aggression, and self-injury.
- A multimodal approach is used in the management of irritability in ASD.
- Individuals with mild irritability may benefit from treatment with an alpha$_2$ adrenergic agonist.
- The atypical antipsychotics are often prescribed for the management of serious behavioral disturbance.
- Risperidone and aripiprazole are the only two Food and Drug Administration–approved medications for irritability in children and adolescents with autism.
- Evidence to date has been mixed regarding the effectiveness of other pharmacologic agents for irritability in ASD.
- Research into the pharmacotherapy of serious behavioral disturbance is needed to develop more effective and better tolerated treatments.

INTRODUCTION

Autism spectrum disorders (ASD) are lifelong neuropsychiatric disorders characterized by impairment in social interaction and communication, as well as repetitive behaviors. The therapeutic approach to the management of ASD is multimodal, often

This work was supported in part by a Daniel X. and Mary Freedman Fellowship in Academic Psychiatry and a Career Development Award (K23 MH 082119) from the National Institute of Mental Health (NIMH).
Disclosure Statement: Dr K.A. Stigler receives research support from Bristol-Myers Squibb, Co, Eli Lilly & Co, Forest Research Institute, Janssen, Novartis, Seaside Therapeutics, and SynapDx.
Department of Psychiatry, Christian Sarkine Autism Treatment Center, Indiana University School of Medicine, Riley Hospital for Children, Room 4300, 705 Riley Hospital Drive, Indianapolis, IN 46202-5200, USA
E-mail address: kstigler@iupui.edu

Child Adolesc Psychiatric Clin N Am 23 (2014) 73–82
http://dx.doi.org/10.1016/j.chc.2013.07.005
1056-4993/14/$ – see front matter © 2014 Elsevier Inc. All rights reserved.

including speech therapy, occupational therapy, social skills training, and physical therapy. In addition to these nonpharmacological treatment modalities, medication is often required to decrease specific target symptoms such as irritability (severe tantrums, aggression, self-injury). Research into the pharmacotherapy of ASD began with the typical antipsychotics in the 1960s. Numerous well-designed studies investigated the high-potency antipsychotic haloperidol, finding the drug effective for serious behavioral disturbance in youth with autism.[1–3] Although beneficial, the drug's potent dopamine D_2 receptor antagonism often led to acute dystonic reactions, as well as drug-induced and withdrawal-related dyskinesias.[4] Concerns regarding the typical antipsychotics led researchers toward the development of the atypical antipsychotics, which has been the most studied drug class in ASD to date. At this time, risperidone and aripiprazole are the only US Food and Drug Administration (FDA)–approved medications to treat irritability in children and adolescents with autism (aged 5–16 years and 6–17 years, respectively). However, in clinical practice, many pharmacologic agents are being prescribed to diminish serious behavioral disturbance in individuals with ASD.

EPIDEMIOLOGY OF ASD

Interfering behavioral problems including irritability, anxiety, and hyperactivity are commonly observed in ASD, with reported prevalence rates of approximately 50% in this population.[5] Furthermore, approximately 30% of individuals with ASD have been shown to exhibit moderate to severe irritability, which left untreated, can significantly impede meaningful participation in behavioral and educational interventions. The management of such behavioral problems frequently necessitates the use of psychotropic medications. In general, pharmacologic agents have been increasingly prescribed for a variety of symptoms in this diagnostic group.[6] This is exemplified by a recent study that examined rates of medication use in 2853 individuals with ASD enrolled in the Autism Treatment Network registry.[6] Among those in the registry, 44% of subjects aged 6 to 11 years and 64% of subjects aged 12 to 17 years, were receiving one or more psychotropic medications.

CURRENT EVIDENCE
Atypical Antipsychotics

Clozapine

To date, 4 small case reports have found clozapine beneficial for symptoms of irritability in children and adults with autism.[7–10] Enuresis, transient sedation, constipation, and sialorrhea were among the adverse effects noted in these reports. Recently, a retrospective medical record review of clozapine was conducted in six patients aged 14 to 34 years with ASD.[11] Significant improvement in aggressive behavior was reported. The drug was considered generally well tolerated. No agranulocytosis was recorded. Constipation, tachycardia, metabolic syndrome, and weight gain (mean weight gain, 14.3 ± 10.9 kg) were reported adverse effects.

Limited research has been conducted on clozapine in ASD for reasons that may include its potential to lower the seizure threshold and its association with agranulocytosis necessitating frequent hematological monitoring.

Risperidone

Risperidone has been investigated for the treatment of irritability in ASD via series, open-label trials, and double-blind, placebo-controlled studies.[12–15] An 8-week, double-blind, placebo-controlled study of risperidone (mean dosage, 1.8 mg/d;

range, 0.5–3.5 mg/d) was conducted in 101 children and adolescents (mean age, 8.8 years) with autism and associated irritability.[15] In this multisite trial, risperidone treatment led to a 57% decrease on the Aberrant Behavior Checklist (ABC) Irritability subscale score versus a 14% reduction with placebo. Furthermore, 69% in the risperidone group, versus 12% in the placebo group, were responders as determined by a rating of "much improved" or "very much improved" on the Clinical Global Impressions-Improvement (CGI-I) scale and a 25% or greater improvement on the ABC Irritability subscale score. Increased appetite, weight gain (risperidone, mean 2.7 kg; placebo, 0.8 kg), dizziness, sedation, and sialorrhea were among the adverse effects reported.

Subjects who responded to risperidone (N = 63) subsequently entered a 16-week, open-label trial.[16] The mean dose of risperidone remained stable during this extension phase. The study participants continued to gain weight, with a mean increase of 5.1 kg over the 24 weeks. After the 16-week phase, 32 subjects considered responders were randomized to either continue risperidone or undergo gradual placebo substitution over 4 weeks. Only 2 (12.5%) of 16 subjects who continued on risperidone were found to relapse. In contrast, 10 (63.5%) of 16 subjects who underwent placebo substitution relapsed, suggesting the need for longer-term treatment.

An 8-week, multisite, double-blind, placebo-controlled study of risperidone (mean dose, 1.2 mg/d) was completed in 79 children and adolescents (mean age, 7.5 years) with ASD.[17] The authors recorded a 64% decrease on the ABC Irritability subscale score with risperidone treatment versus a 31% reduction with placebo. In addition, 53% of subjects in the risperidone group were deemed responders in comparison to 18% of those in the placebo group. Adverse effects included sedation, tachycardia, extrapyramidal symptoms (EPS), increased appetite, and weight gain (risperidone, 2.7 kg; placebo, 1 kg), among others.

Randomized controlled trials of risperidone have also been conducted in young children with ASD. A double-blind, placebo-controlled trial of risperidone was completed in 40 children (age range, 2–9 years) over a duration of 6 months.[18] Risperidone at a total daily dose of 1 mg/d was considered efficacious for symptoms of hyperactivity and aggression. Adverse effects included sedation, transient dyskinesia, increased appetite, and weight gain (risperidone, 2.8 kg; placebo, 1.7 kg).

Another placebo-controlled study of risperidone (mean dose, 1.1 mg/d; range, 0.5–1.5 mg/d) in 24 children (age range, 2–6 years) with ASD found the drug minimally efficacious in comparison to placebo; possibly because study participation did not require high levels of baseline irritability.[19] Transient sedation, sialorrhea, and weight gain (risperidone, 3 kg; placebo, 0.6 kg) were among the adverse effects reported.

Olanzapine

A 12-week, open-label study of olanzapine (mean dose, 7.8 mg/d) in ASD found six (86%) of seven study completers (mean age, 20.9 years; range, 5–42 years) responded to the drug.[20] Although symptoms such as irritability and hyperactivity improved, subjects experienced adverse effects including sedation, increased appetite, and weight gain (mean, 8.4 kg). A 6-week, open-label study of olanzapine (mean dose, 7.9 mg/d) was completed in 12 children with autism (mean age, 7.8 years), using haloperidol (mean dose, 1.4 mg/d) as a standard comparator.[21] Five (83%) of six subjects were considered responders in the olanzapine group and three (50%) of six subjects were deemed responders in the haloperidol group. On average, olanzapine treatment (mean, 4.1 kg; range, 2.7–7.2 kg) was associated with greater weight gain versus haloperidol treatment (mean, 1.4 kg; range, −2.5 to +4 kg). A small 8-week, double-blind, placebo-controlled trial of olanzapine (mean dose, 10 mg/d; range, 7.5–12.5 mg/d) was conducted in 11 youth with ASD (age range, 6–14 years).[22] Three (50%) of six subjects in the olanzapine group were judged responders, compared with one (20%) of five subjects in the placebo group. Adverse effects included sedation, increased appetite, and weight gain (olanzapine, 3.4 kg; placebo, 0.68 kg).

Quetiapine

Retrospective and open-label studies of quetiapine have been published in ASD, with mixed findings. A retrospective medical record review of quetiapine (mean dose, 249 mg/d; range, 25–600 mg/d) found that 8 (40%) of 20 patients with ASD (mean age, 12.1 years; range, 5–28 years) responded to the drug over a mean duration of 60 weeks (range, 4–180 weeks).[23] Adverse effects were recorded in half of the patients and resulted in drug discontinuation in 15%. Another retrospective review of quetiapine (mean dose, 477 mg/d) was conducted in 10 subjects (age range, 5–19 years) with ASD over a mean duration of 22 weeks (range, 10–48 weeks).[24] The authors reported that 6 (60%) of 10 patients responded to the drug, with improvement noted in symptoms of hyperactivity and inattention. Mild sedation, weight gain, and sialorrhea were among the adverse effects recorded.

A small 16-week, open-label study of quetiapine (mean dose, 225 mg/d) in six subjects (mean age, 10.9 years; range, 6–15 years) with autism found that only two (33%) youth responded to the drug.[25] Of the other four subjects, three withdrew because of sedation or lack of effectiveness, and one withdrew due to a possible seizure. Behavioral activation, increased appetite, and weight gain (range, 0.9–8.2 kg) were also noted. Another small open-label study of quetiapine (mean dose, 292 mg/d; range, 100–450 mg/d) was completed in nine subjects with autism aged 10 to 17 years (mean age, 14.6 years).[26] In this 12-week study, two participants (22%) were considered responders. Two subjects withdrew from the study due to sedation or agitation and aggression. Commonly reported adverse effects included sedation, weight gain, and increased agitation.

Ziprasidone

Ziprasidone (mean dose, 59.2 mg/d; range, 20–120 mg/d) was investigated in 12 youth (mean age, 11.6 years; range, 8–20 years) with autism or pervasive developmental disorder not otherwise specified.[27] This case series found 6 (50%) of 12 subjects responded to the drug over a mean treatment duration of 14.2 weeks (range, 6–30 weeks). Improvement was observed in symptoms of aggression, agitation, and irritability. Transient sedation was the most commonly reported adverse effect. There were no reported cardiovascular adverse effects. A mean change in weight of −2.6 kg (range, −16 to +2.7 kg) was recorded.

A 6-week, open-label study of ziprasidone was completed in 12 adolescents, aged 12 to 18 years (range, 14.5 years), with autism and associated irritability.[28] The study found that 9 (75%) of 12 subjects responded to the drug at a mean dosage of 98.3 mg/d (range, 20–160 mg/d). Sedation was a commonly reported adverse effect. Dystonic reactions developed in two study participants. Ziprasidone treatment was weight neutral and led to decreased measures of total cholesterol. The mean QTc at study endpoint increased by 14.7 ms.

The association of ziprasidone with QTc prolongation on electrocardiography resulted in an FDA warning. Individuals with known cardiac disease (eg, cardiac arrhythmias, long QT syndrome) or those taking other drugs that can prolong the QTc interval should not be prescribed ziprasidone without careful monitoring and consultation with a cardiologist.

Aripiprazole

Case series, open-label studies, and double-blind, placebo-controlled trials have found aripiprazole effective for the treatment of irritability in ASD.[29–31] An 8-week, double-blind, placebo-controlled, fixed-dose study of aripiprazole was conducted in 231 children and adolescents (age range, 6–17 years) with autism.[30] In this study, participants received placebo or aripiprazole (5, 10, or 15 mg/d). Significant improvement in symptoms of irritability was found at all doses of the drug, as measured by the ABC Irritability subscale score. However, only the 5 mg/d treatment group responded to aripiprazole, based on a CGI-I scale score of "much improved" or "very much improved" and a 25% or greater improvement on the ABC Irritability subscale score. Sedation, EPS, and weight gain were among the adverse effects reported. Serious adverse events included presyncope (N = 1) and increased aggression (N = 1).

Another 8-week, double-blind, placebo-controlled trial of aripiprazole in 98 youth (age range, 6–17 years) with autism used a flexible dosing schedule (2–15 mg/d).[31] Significant improvement in irritability was recorded, as determined by the ABC Irritability subscale score. In addition, significantly more subjects in the aripiprazole group, versus the placebo group, were considered responders, as measured by a rating of "much improved" or "very much improved" on the CGI-I scale and a 25% or greater improvement on the ABC Irritability subscale score. Adverse effects included sedation, vomiting, drooling, tremor, and weight gain, among others.

A subsequent 52-week, open-label study of aripiprazole (dose range, 2–15 mg/d) investigated the drug's long-term safety and tolerability in 300 subjects aged 6 to 17 years with autism.[32] The study included de novo subjects as well as participants of the aforementioned double-blind studies.[30,31] Concomitant psychotropic medications (except alpha-2 agonists, carbamazepine, oxcarbazepine, and other antipsychotics) were allowed during the trial. A total of 199 (60%) of 300 subjects completed the trial, with the authors concluding that aripiprazole was generally safe and well tolerated. Increased appetite, weight gain, vomiting, and insomnia were among the more commonly reported adverse effects. A secondary paper that evaluated the drug's effectiveness found most subjects "much" or "very much" improved on the CGI-I at study endpoint.[33] Overall, the study concluded that aripiprazole decreased irritability for up to a year in children and adolescents with autism.

Paliperidone

Paliperidone was investigated in an 8-week, open-label study of 25 adolescents and young adults (mean age, 15.3 years; range, 12–21 years) with autism.[34] The investigators found that 21 (84%) of the subjects responded to paliperidone at a mean dose of 7.1 mg/d (range, 3–12 mg/d), as determined by a CGI-I scale score of "much improved" or "very much improved" and a 25% or greater improvement on the ABC Irritability subscale score. Participants, on average, gained 2.2 kg (range, −3.6 to +7.9 kg) during the trial. Although mean serum prolactin increased over the 8 weeks [5.3 ng/mL (baseline); 41.4 (endpoint)], no signs or symptoms of hyperprolactinemia were recorded. Other adverse effects included sedation, EPS, and increased appetite.

Alpha$_2$ Adrenergic Agonists

Clonidine

A small 6-week, double-blind, placebo-controlled, crossover study of clonidine (4–10 μg/kg/d) in eight youth with autism (mean age, 8.1 years; range, 5–13 years) found disparate results.[35] Although parent and teacher ratings noted significant improvement in irritability, hyperactivity, and oppositionality with clonidine versus placebo, investigator ratings found no significant difference between treatment groups. Sedation, hypotension, and decreased activity were among the adverse effects recorded. A 4-week, double-blind, placebo-controlled, crossover study of transdermal clonidine (mean dosage, 3.6 μg/kg/d; range, 0.16–0.48 mg/d) was conducted in nine subjects with autism (mean age, 12.9 years; range, 5–33 years).[36] Symptoms of impulsivity and hyperactivity were noted to improve with clonidine. Sedation and fatigue were among the adverse effects reported.

Guanfacine

An 8-week, prospective, open-label trial of guanfacine (dose range, 1–3 mg/d) recorded improvement in hyperactivity in 12 (48%) of 25 subjects with ASD.[37] Parent ratings also noted a significant reduction in symptoms of irritability. The study participants (mean age, 9 years; range, 5–14 years) were previous nonresponders to methylphenidate. Adverse effects included irritability, sedation, and sleep disturbance. Three subjects discontinued study participation due to decreased frustration tolerance and tearfulness.

A 6-week, double-blind, placebo-controlled, crossover study of guanfacine (dose range, 1–3 mg/d) was conducted in 11 children (mean age, 7.3 years; range, 5–9 years) with intellectual disability and/or an ASD.[38] A significant reduction in hyperactivity was found in 45% of the subjects. However, no significant improvement was observed in symptoms of irritability. Sedation and increased irritability were among the adverse effects recorded.

Mood Stabilizers and Anticonvulsants

Lithium

A case report described lithium (900 mg/d) augmentation of fluvoxamine treatment in an adult with autism.[39] The authors noted improvement in aggression and impulsivity after 2 weeks of treatment.

Divalproex sodium

Open-label and double-blind, placebo-controlled studies have investigated divalproex sodium in ASD.[40–42] An 8-week, double-blind, placebo-controlled trial of divalproex sodium (mean endpoint blood level, 77.8 μg/mL) for irritability was completed in 30 subjects (age range, 6–20 years) with ASD.[42] The authors found no significant difference between drug and placebo, as determined by the ABC Irritability subscale. Increased appetite, hyperammonemia, and skin rash requiring study discontinuation were among the adverse effects recorded. Divalproex sodium was also investigated in a 12-week, double-blind, placebo-controlled study of 27 children and adolescents (age range, 5–15 years) with ASD and irritability.[41] In this study, 62.5% of subjects in the divalproex sodium group [mean blood level, 89.8 μg/mL (responders); 64.3 μg/mL (nonresponders)], compared with 9% in the placebo group, were considered responders. Adverse effects included weight gain, headache, and insomnia, among others.

Lamotrigine

A 12-week, double-blind, placebo-controlled trial of lamotrigine (5 mg/kg/d) was conducted in 28 children (mean age, 5.8 years; range, 3–11 years) with autism.[43] No significant difference was found between the drug and placebo groups as based on several rating scales, including the ABC Irritability subscale score. The most frequently reported adverse effects were insomnia and hyperactivity.

Levetiracetam

A 10-week, double-blind, placebo-controlled trial of levetiracetam (mean dose, 862.5 mg/d) in 20 youth (age range, 5–17 years) with autism found no significant difference between drug and placebo on measures assessing aggression and affective instability.[44] Aggression, agitation, and hyperactivity were among the recorded adverse effects.

DISCUSSION

Most evidence to date supports the use of atypical antipsychotics as first-line pharmacotherapeutic agents for targeting irritability in ASD. As such, risperidone and aripiprazole are the only drugs currently approved for this target symptom domain in children and adolescents with autism. Relatively small controlled studies of the anticonvulsants and mood stabilizers for irritability in youth with ASD have generally demonstrated negative results. Ongoing large-scale controlled studies of medications such as guanfacine may shed light on the usefulness of alpha$_2$ adrenergic agonists for symptoms of milder irritability in this population.

CONCLUSION AND FUTURE DIRECTIONS

Research into the pharmacotherapy of severe behavioral disturbance in ASD has primarily focused on the atypical antipsychotics. Although these studies have significantly contributed to the pharmacologic management of this symptom domain in ASD, there remains an ongoing need to identify more effective and better tolerated treatments in this population. Compounds with different mechanisms of action will continue to be explored. As such, one recent study investigated the use of the glutamatergic modulator and antioxidant N-acetylcysteine for irritability in 33 children (age range, 3–10 years) with autism.[45] In this 12-week, double-blind, placebo-controlled trial, the drug dosage was increased by 900 mg/d every 4 weeks to reach a final target dose of 900 mg three times daily. Subjects in the N-acetylcysteine group, compared to the placebo group, demonstrated significant improvement in irritability as measured by the ABC Irritability subscale. The drug was generally well tolerated. Although these findings are encouraging, the severity of irritability at baseline (mean ABC Irritability subscale score = 17) was notably lower than that of studies of risperidone and aripiprazole (mean ABC Irritability subscale score = 26 and 28, respectively).[15,30] Additional research is needed to better understand the potential role of N-acetylcysteine, as well as other novel compounds, in the treatment of irritability in ASD.

REFERENCES

1. Campbell M, Anderson LT, Meier M, et al. A comparison of haloperidol and behavior therapy and their interaction in autistic children. J Am Acad Child Psychiatry 1978;17(4):640–55.
2. Perry R, Campbell M, Adams P, et al. Long-term efficacy of haloperidol in autistic children: continuous versus discontinuous drug administration. J Am Acad Child Adolesc Psychiatry 1989;28(1):87–92.
3. Cohen IL, Campbell M, Posner D, et al. Behavioral effects of haloperidol in young autistic children. An objective analysis using a within-subjects reversal design. J Am Acad Child Psychiatry 1980;19(4):665–77.
4. Campbell M, Armenteros JL, Malone RP, et al. Neuroleptic-related dyskinesias in autistic children: a prospective, longitudinal study. J Am Acad Child Adolesc Psychiatry 1997;36(6):835–43.

5. Lecavalier L. Behavioral and emotional problems in young people with pervasive developmental disorders: relative prevalence, effects of subject characteristics, and empirical classification. J Autism Dev Disord 2006;36(8): 1101–14.

6. Coury DL, Anagnostou E, Manning-Courtney P, et al. Use of psychotropic medication in children and adolescents with autism spectrum disorders. Pediatrics 2012;130(Suppl 2):S69–76.

7. Zuddas A, Ledda MG, Fratta A, et al. Clinical effects of clozapine on autistic disorder. Am J Psychiatry 1996;153(5):738.

8. Chen NC, Bedair HS, McKay B, et al. Clozapine in the treatment of aggression in an adolescent with autistic disorder. J Clin Psychiatry 2001;62(6):479–80.

9. Gobbi G, Pulvirenti L. Long-term treatment with clozapine in an adult with autistic disorder accompanied by aggressive behaviour. J Psychiatry Neurosci 2001; 26(4):340–1.

10. Lambrey S, Falissard B, Martin-Barrero M, et al. Effectiveness of clozapine for the treatment of aggression in an adolescent with autistic disorder. J Child Adolesc Psychopharmacol 2010;20(1):79–80.

11. Beherec L, Lambrey S, Quilici G, et al. Retrospective review of clozapine in the treatment of patients with autism spectrum disorder and severe disruptive behaviors. J Clin Psychopharmacol 2011;31(3):341–4.

12. McDougle CJ, Holmes JP, Bronson MR, et al. Risperidone treatment of children and adolescents with pervasive developmental disorders: a prospective open-label study. J Am Acad Child Adolesc Psychiatry 1997;36(5):685–93.

13. Findling RL, Maxwell K, Wiznitzer M. An open clinical trial of risperidone monotherapy in young children with autistic disorder. Psychopharmacol Bull 1997; 33(1):155–9.

14. Nicolson R, Awad G, Sloman L. An open trial of risperidone in young autistic children. J Am Acad Child Adolesc Psychiatry 1998;37(4):372–6.

15. Research Units on Pediatric Psychopharmacology, Autism Network. Risperidone in children with autism and serious behavioral problems. N Engl J Med 2002; 347(5):314–21.

16. Research Units on Pediatric Psychopharmacology Autism Network. Risperidone treatment of autistic disorder: longer-term benefits and blinded discontinuation after 6 months. Am J Psychiatry 2005;162(7):1361–9.

17. Shea S, Turgay A, Carroll A, et al. Risperidone in the treatment of disruptive behavioral symptoms in children with autistic and other pervasive developmental disorders. Pediatrics 2004;114(5):e634–41.

18. Nagaraj R, Singhi P, Malhi P. Risperidone in children with autism: randomized, placebo-controlled, double-blind study. J Child Neurol 2006;21(6):450–5.

19. Luby J, Mrakotsky C, Stalets MM, et al. Risperidone in preschool children with autistic spectrum disorders: an investigation of safety and efficacy. J Child Adolesc Psychopharmacol 2006;16(5):575–87.

20. Potenza MN, Holmes JP, Kanes SJ, et al. Olanzapine treatment of children, adolescents, and adults with pervasive developmental disorders: an open-label pilot study. J Clin Psychopharmacol 1999;19(1):37–44.

21. Malone RP, Cater J, Sheikh RM, et al. Olanzapine versus haloperidol in children with autistic disorder: an open pilot study. J Am Acad Child Adolesc Psychiatry 2001;40(8):887–94.

22. Hollander E, Wasserman S, Swanson EN, et al. A double-blind placebo-controlled pilot study of olanzapine in childhood/adolescent pervasive developmental disorder. J Child Adolesc Psychopharmacol 2006;16(5):541–8.

23. Corson AH, Barkenbus JE, Posey DJ, et al. A retrospective analysis of quetiapine in the treatment of pervasive developmental disorders. J Clin Psychiatry 2004; 65(11):1531–6.

24. Hardan AY, Jou RJ, Handen BL. Retrospective study of quetiapine in children and adolescents with pervasive developmental disorders. J Autism Dev Disord 2005; 35(3):387–91.

25. Martin A, Koenig K, Scahill L, et al. Open-label quetiapine in the treatment of children and adolescents with autistic disorder. J Child Adolesc Psychopharmacol 1999;9(2):99–107.

26. Findling RL, McNamara NK, Gracious BL, et al. Quetiapine in nine youths with autistic disorder. J Child Adolesc Psychopharmacol 2004;14(2):287–94.

27. McDougle CJ, Kem DL, Posey DJ. Case series: use of ziprasidone for maladaptive symptoms in youths with autism. J Am Acad Child Adolesc Psychiatry 2002; 41(8):921–7.

28. Malone RP, Delaney MA, Hyman SB, et al. Ziprasidone in adolescents with autism: an open-label pilot study. J Child Adolesc Psychopharmacol 2007; 17(6):779–90.

29. Stigler KA, Diener JT, Kohn AE, et al. Aripiprazole in pervasive developmental disorder not otherwise specified and Asperger's disorder: a 14-week, prospective, open-label study. J Child Adolesc Psychopharmacol 2009;19(3):265–74.

30. Marcus RN, Owen R, Kamen L, et al. A placebo-controlled, fixed-dose study of aripiprazole in children and adolescents with irritability associated with autistic disorder. J Am Acad Child Adolesc Psychiatry 2009;48(11):1110–9.

31. Owen R, Sikich L, Marcus RN, et al. Aripiprazole in the treatment of irritability in children and adolescents with autistic disorder. Pediatrics 2009;124(6): 1533–40.

32. Marcus RN, Owen R, Manos G, et al. Safety and tolerability of aripiprazole for irritability in pediatric patients with autistic disorder: a 52-week, open-label, multicenter study. J Clin Psychiatry 2011;72(9):1270–6.

33. Marcus RN, Owen R, Manos G, et al. Aripiprazole in the treatment of irritability in pediatric patients (aged 6-17 years) with autistic disorder: results from a 52-week, open-label study. J Child Adolesc Psychopharmacol 2011;21(3):229–36.

34. Stigler KA, Mullett JE, Erickson CA, et al. Paliperidone for irritability in adolescents and young adults with autistic disorder. Psychopharmacology (Berl) 2012;223(2):237–45.

35. Jaselskis CA, Cook EH Jr, Fletcher KE, et al. Clonidine treatment of hyperactive and impulsive children with autistic disorder. J Clin Psychopharmacol 1992; 12(5):322–7.

36. Fankhauser MP, Karumanchi VC, German ML, et al. A double-blind, placebo-controlled study of the efficacy of transdermal clonidine in autism. J Clin Psychiatry 1992;53(3):77–82.

37. Scahill L, Aman MG, McDougle CJ, et al. A prospective open trial of guanfacine in children with pervasive developmental disorders. J Child Adolesc Psychopharmacol 2006;16(5):589–98.

38. Handen BL, Sahl R, Hardan AY. Guanfacine in children with autism and/or intellectual disabilities. J Dev Behav Pediatr 2008;29(4):303–8.

39. Epperson CN, McDougle CJ, Anand A, et al. Lithium augmentation of fluvoxamine in autistic disorder: a case report. J Child Adolesc Psychopharmacol 1994;4(3):201–7.

40. Hollander E, Dolgoff-Kaspar R, Cartwright C, et al. An open trial of divalproex sodium in autism spectrum disorders. J Clin Psychiatry 2001;62(7):530–4.

41. Hollander E, Chaplin W, Soorya L, et al. Divalproex sodium vs placebo for the treatment of irritability in children and adolescents with autism spectrum disorders. Neuropsychopharmacology 2010;35(4):990–8.
42. Hellings JA, Weckbaugh M, Nickel EJ, et al. A double-blind, placebo-controlled study of valproate for aggression in youth with pervasive developmental disorders. J Child Adolesc Psychopharmacol 2005;15(4):682–92.
43. Belsito KM, Law PA, Kirk KS, et al. Lamotrigine therapy for autistic disorder: a randomized, double-blind, placebo-controlled trial. J Autism Dev Disord 2001;31(2): 175–81.
44. Wasserman S, Iyengar R, Chaplin WF, et al. Levetiracetam versus placebo in childhood and adolescent autism: a double-blind placebo-controlled study. Clin Psychopharmacol 2006;21(6):363–7.
45. Hardan AY, Fung LK, Libove RA, et al. A randomized controlled pilot trial of oral N-acetylcysteine in children with autism. Biol Psychiatry 2012;71(11):956–61.

Management of Agitation in Individuals with Autism Spectrum Disorders in the Emergency Department

John J. McGonigle, PhD[a],*, Arvind Venkat, MD[b],
Carol Beresford, MD[c], Thomas P. Campbell, MD, MPH[b],
Robin L. Gabriels, PsyD[c]

KEYWORDS

- Autism spectrum disorders • Emergency department • Crisis management
- Acute agitation • Emergency evaluation and treatment
- Least-restrictive treatment model • Restraint

KEY POINTS

- Medical and psychiatric causes of agitation in patients with autism spectrum disorder (ASD) in the emergency department (ED).
- Rapid assessment of acute agitation.
- Nonpharmacologic and behavioral interventions in the ED.
- Reducing agitation by adapting care and treatment around the core features of ASD.
- Use of psychiatric and psychoactive medications in EDs for treating acute agitation in patients with ASD.
- Restraint and seclusion for agitated patients with ASD in the ED.

OVERVIEW

Individuals with autism spectrum disorders (ASD) presenting with acute agitation, including dangerous behaviors to self and others, often cause families, caregivers, educators, and first responders to turn to the hospital emergency department (ED) in times of crisis. An additional challenge for medical and psychiatric hospital

Disclosure Statement: None.
[a] Western Psychiatric Institute and Clinic of UPMC, University of Pittsburgh, School of Medicine, 3811 O'Hara Street, Pittsburgh, PA 15213, USA; [b] Department of Emergency Medicine, West Penn Allegheny Health System, 320 East North Avenue, Pittsburgh, PA 15212, USA; [c] Department of Psychiatry, University of Colorado Denver, Children's Hospital Colorado, 13123 East 16th Avenue, Aurora, CO 80045, USA
* Corresponding author.
E-mail address: mcgoniglejj@upmc.edu

personnel in the ED setting is teasing out the core deficits of ASD (social-communication and restricted and repetitive behavior patterns and interests) from acute underlying medical and/or psychiatric conditions. This article presents a framework for improving the crisis evaluation of the tip-of-the-iceberg presenting behaviors of individuals with ASD and provides a suggested least-restrictive treatment model for adapting the ED environment to improve the care of these patients.

INTRODUCTION

Individuals with ASD can present challenging behaviors and agitation. These behaviors can be dangerous, creating stress and difficulty for families, caregivers, educators, and first responders, leading to the presentation of these individuals to the hospital ED.[1] Acute management and de-escalation of children, adolescents, and adults with ASD has had limited success and has often resulted in unwanted outcomes.[2,3] The results of a 2011 survey in Pennsylvania of 3500 children, adolescents, and adults with ASD found that 28% of the respondents who required an ED or hospital evaluation for behavioral/psychiatric or medical reasons had negative experiences and unwanted outcomes.[4] The lack of communication, education, and experience of the ED personnel evaluating and treating individuals with ASD may contribute to the prevalence of these negative experiences. This lack of training causes difficulty in differentiating ASD diagnostic features from the onset of acute medical or psychiatric symptoms.

Symptoms of ASD

The presence of the core communication and social impairments unique to the ASD population complicates their behavioral, psychiatric, and medical management. Specifically, ASD represents a class of life-long neurodevelopmental disorders characterized by impairments in reciprocal social interactions; communication skills; and restricted, repetitive, and stereotyped patterns of behavior, interests, and activities.[5] In addition to these core diagnostic features, a range of other nonspecific atypical behaviors, such as anxiety, depression, sleeping and eating disturbances, attention issues, temper tantrums, and aggression or self-injury, are common. It has been found that features of ASD are often accompanied by impairments in cognitive and adaptive functioning, learning styles, attention skills, and sensory processing abilities.[6] Gabriels[7] (2011) reviewed the ASD diagnostic and associated issues that can affect presenting behaviors in children, adolescents, and adults with ASD.[7] For example, individuals with ASD generally have a unique pattern of markedly low adaptive functioning levels even though their intelligence levels may be higher compared with their levels of adaptive functioning.

Individuals with ASD display great variability in the range and severity of the core diagnostic features.[5] For example, some individuals may isolate themselves because of their focus on engaging in their own restricted interests or repetitive behaviors, whereas others may seem social but are odd or inappropriate in their social approaches to others and unaware of the impact of their behaviors on others. Behavioral expressions of ASD will also vary. Some individuals with an ASD may engage in stereotyped and repetitive body movements, manipulation of object parts, or self-injurious behaviors, whereas others are preoccupied with compulsive or ritualized behaviors, have a rigid insistence on sameness of the environment, or engage in circumscribed interests. Finally, individuals with ASD may also display a variety of associated impairments in intelligence and adaptive abilities, comorbid medical and psychiatric diagnoses, and sensory sensitivities, all of which can complicate the evaluation of presenting crisis behaviors seen in an ED setting.[8–11]

Atypical responses to sensory input (eg, over-responsiveness and/or under-responsiveness) in individuals with ASD have been reported in numerous studies.[12,13] Individuals with ASD tend to be very distractible and can be abnormally aroused or distracted by sensory input, such as sound, touch, smell, taste, or movement.[14,15] These abnormal sensory responses to stimuli can make some experiences in unfamiliar settings (eg, hospital settings) intolerable to the child with ASD, causing them to display tantrums or other symptoms of distress (eg, self-injury or aggression). Given the fact that patients with ASD can be extremely sensitive to environmental stimuli and unpredictability, these individuals depend on routines and continuity. Thus, they may respond best if given a place to retreat and isolate as opposed to being further agitated. Unfamiliar settings or procedures can cause anxiety, which they may express through disruptive or aggressive behaviors because of their social-communication skill limitations. Intellectual and communication impairments can contribute to these individuals' inability to understand expectations. These impairments may limit their ability to report internal physical or emotional experiences, which is often expected of children and adolescents in order to complete successful psychiatric assessments or medical examinations. Given these impairments, children and adolescents with an ASD are not likely to respond positively to intervention strategies (eg, verbal reassurance, coaxing, or explanations) that are typically used by ED personnel with children who have a capacity for insight and reciprocal social-communication exchanges.

Given that 1 in 88 children are now being identified with ASD[16] along with the increase in hospitalization rates of patients with ASD (particularly those aged 7–12 years),[17] ED personnel and crisis responders need to understand the unique needs of individuals with ASD. This understanding will allow acute care personnel to rapidly assess and optimize effective treatment that is delivered in a least-restrictive manner in the ED setting. Psychiatric disorders are common in children with ASD who often have comorbid conditions. In 2008, Simonoff and colleagues[18] conducted a study of 112 adolescents between 10 and 14 years of age with ASD through parent interviews and using the Child and Adolescent Psychiatric Assessment and found that 70% of the participants had at least one comorbid psychiatric condition (social anxiety, attention-deficit/hyperactivity disorder, oppositional defiant disorder) and as many as 41% of the patients have at least 2 comorbid conditions.[18]

The purpose of this article is to describe the challenges that individuals with ASD face in receiving treatment in crisis and emergency situations. Additionally, this article provides information for emergency physicians, ED personnel, and crisis response teams on a systematic, least-restrictive approach when assessing and providing treatment of acute agitation to patients with ASD in crisis and ED settings.

RAPID ASSESSMENT OF CRISIS BEHAVIORS IN INDIVIDUALS WITH ASD

Given the core features of ASD, the challenge for emergency medical personnel is to systematically gather the key information necessary to address the issues that may be underlying or contributing to the tip-of-the-iceberg crisis behavior presentation of individuals with ASD. (See Gabriels[7] for an extensive review of issues unique to the ASD population than can affect behavioral presentations.) The *tip of the iceberg* refers to some of the observable signs of acute agitation with the underlying causes beneath the surface. Beginning with an assessment framework that focuses on considering what may be driving the crisis behaviors has the advantage of efficiently targeting and addressing the behavior problems. For example, a sudden onset of behavioral and emotional disturbance can indicate the possibility of a medical illness. Crying from pain is often difficult to distinguish from that caused by anxiety.[19]

Initial Assessment Interview

It is suggested that an initial interview with the caregivers of individuals with ASD begin with gathering details of the presenting crisis behaviors to aid in the development of a plan for medical and/or psychiatric tests and interventions. Beginning questions should include the following: (1) What are the presenting crisis behaviors? (2) Are these behaviors a *change* from the typical ASD symptom presentation? (3) In what way have the crisis behaviors changed? (Are the crisis behaviors new for the individual or do the crisis behaviors represent a deterioration or escalation of long-standing existing behaviors?) (4) In what situations do these behaviors usually occur (antecedents)? (5) What are the typical responses or (consequences) given when these behaviors are observed?

The responses to these initial questions will then lead the interviewer to the next step of gathering information in key areas that may be contributing factors (ie, medical, psychiatric, sensory issues, communication skills, social skills, motor skills, cognitive/academic issues, and family/community environment issues).

Medical Issues

There are many medical issues to consider: constipation related to being on certain medications or having poor nutrition (including pica); seizures (In the ASD population, there is a 25%–33% risk of seizures, and those at a higher risk are children younger than 5 years of age) children entering puberty[11]; and individuals with more severe cognitive, motor, and language impairments.[20] Other individuals at risk include those with ear infections, dental infection, pain issues resulting from poor dental hygiene or care, sleep problems (Poor quality, of sleep in the ASD population seems to be related to exacerbated behavioral symptoms.),[21] undetected injuries, sleep apnea, or urinary tract infections. Other medical issues that were identified in a sample of 151 patients with ASD aged 4 to 17 years admitted to a specialized psychiatric hospital unit included headaches, gastroesophageal reflux disease, obesity, hypothyroidism, enuresis, encopresis, asthma, hyperlipidemia, hearing loss, traumatic brain injury, tuberous sclerosis, sex chromosome abnormalities, Prader Willi syndrome, and juvenile rheumatoid arthritis.[22]

Psychiatric Issues

In the ASD population, high rates of affective (depression) and anxiety disorders have been reported.[18,23] Additionally, affective disorders tend to peak in adolescence and young adulthood and can be signaled by deteriorating behaviors.[24]

Sensory and Self-regulation Issues

Individuals with ASD can be abnormally aroused or distracted by sensory input, such as sound, touch, smell, taste, or movement. Individuals with ASD may have been exposed to a decrease in sensory stimuli or an increase in chaos within their community environments causing them to respond in order to seek out or retreat from the sensory input in a potentially inappropriate or dangerous manner.[13,15]

Communication Issues

Does the individual have significant problems with verbal expression or does he or she use other means of communication, such as the use of pictures or signs to communicate. Have the communication strategies/abilities of the individual decreased recently?

Social Skills Deficit

An example might include the following scenario: A patient has autism and has difficulty with turn taking and following social cues, it is important to consider if the patient is being bullied at school or may be displaying dangerous, suicidal, or aggressive behaviors.

Motor Skills Deficit

Has the individual shown a decrease in their motor strength and motor coordination (eg, has a hard time with buttons and tying shoelaces when not previously observed).

Academic/Cognitive/Adaptive Skill Deficit

Is there an underlying learning disability that may or may not have been evaluated by IQ and achievement testing? Has the individual shown a decline in their self-care skills, including toileting issues? For example, is the patient smearing feces now or wetting the bed, which can then indicate the possible onset of a psychiatric, medical, or trauma/abuse issue?

Family/Community Environment

Has there been a significant change in the family circumstances of the patient (eg, parents divorced and each now have new partners and step children or divorce with shuttling of the patient between different living environments)?

INITIAL MEDICAL EVALUATION OF PATIENTS WITH ASD WITH ACUTE AGITATION

Following the initial interview, the next step is to rule out or address any medical factors that may be contributing to the presenting symptoms. Agitation is typically defined as a state of chronic restlessness with increased psychomotor activity generally observed as an expression of emotional tension and characterized by purposeless, restless activity.[25] Pacing, talking, crying, and laughing sometimes are characteristics and may serve to release nervous tension associated with anxiety, fear, or other mental stress. For individuals with ASD, these symptoms are often expressed in atypical and unusual ways. In considering how to treat agitation in patients with ASD, it is imperative to determine whether there is an underlying medical cause to the change in behavior that requires intervention. In all cases, it is acceptable to presume that there is a medical cause of acute agitation that is perceived as a change in behavior by the caregiver until proven otherwise. For patients presenting to the ED, there are initial historical and physical examination factors that will indicate that a medical cause of agitation is likely. Abnormal vital signs, including extremes (high or low) of pulse, blood pressure, respiratory rate, oxygenation, temperature, and blood sugar, should raise a high suspicion that agitation is not caused by a primary psychiatric cause. Historical factors that also point to nonbehavioral causes of agitation include reports of memory loss, acute delirium, headache (especially if coupled with focal neurologic deficits or seizures), increased muscle tone or weakness, temperature intolerance, and overt signs of trauma and psychosis without previous psychiatric history. Physical examination findings that suggest a medical cause of agitation include unequal pupils, decreased coordination, and slurred speech. The presence of any of these factors should lead to an emergent medical evaluation of causes of agitation.[26] For patients with ASD, impairments in communication and social interaction may pose specific challenges to assessing whether any of these history or physical examination findings are present. Reliance on techniques suggested by the caregiver may allow a more accurate assessment of the history and physical examination. Dietary habits, both in terms of type and timing of oral intake, can reveal whether patients may be at risk for gastrointestinal causes of acute agitation, such as constipation. Understanding whether any changes have been made in the pharmacologic management of the patients may reveal possible side effects of medication that may be causing acute behavioral changes. Similarly, knowledge of vaccination and menstrual history may provide insight as to whether an infectious disease or experiencing pain that cannot be easily expressed may be causing agitation. Finally, knowledge of the sleep pattern and acute changes therein may point to insomnia as a cause of agitation.[27]

Medical Causes of Agitation in Patients with Autism

Although autism has been primarily treated as a neurodevelopmental disorder, there is an increasing understanding that medical comorbidities are often present in individuals with autism[24]; understanding where there is an intersection between these conditions and acute agitation can allow a more effective assessment and treatment. The common association between autism and seizures should also lead to a careful assessment of whether agitation in patients is caused by seizure activity. The combination of change in sleep habits with agitation may suggest that behavioral changes are caused by seizures that are affecting normal sleep hygiene. A careful history from the caregiver of agitation following unusual patterns of thrashing or convulsions may suggest seizure activity.[28]

Catatonia is a medical emergency that may cause an acute change in behavior in patients with autism. A complaint from the caregiver of a loss of the ability to perform activities of daily living, food refusal, a slowing of speech, and a change in interactions with the environment should lead to a more in-depth evaluation of whether catatonia may be present. Finally, self-injurious behavior may lead to injuries of the head, face, and hands. A careful physical examination may allow the diagnosis of such injuries as the cause of agitation in patients with ASD.[27]

USE OF PSYCHOTROPIC MEDICATIONS IN ED

The pharmacologic management of acute agitation of patients with autism in the ED is a vital adjunct to appropriate care in this setting. Therapeutic communication using verbal de-escalation techniques of any agitated patient is always preferable for the safety of the patient and staff, but medication may be needed.[29,30] Parents or caregivers can be helpful resources because they are experts in the stimuli that may increase or decrease agitation. It is always prudent to ask the parents or caregivers about a previous need for medications to reduce anxiety or agitation and the patients' previous response.[31] It is also important to educate parents, caregivers, and support staff about all of the processes and decisions that may need to be made so they can assist and advocate for patients. This sharing of information will require planning and patience to avoid frustration. The risk and benefit of using pharmacologic means to reduce agitation should always be weighed and discussed with parents, caregivers, and guardians. If available, dedicated psychiatric EDs are an important part of the array of treatments for children and adolescents with ASD who present with acute agitation or a behavioral emergency.

The use of medication is an important adjunct toward the goal of calming children or adults with ASD, after efforts to provide an appropriately structured and soothing environment as well as attempts at verbal de-escalation. The same medications that are used for adults with ASD in psychiatric EDs are the same as those used for children. These medications include benzodiazepines and antipsychotics. Many patients with autism have other diseases that may complicate the choice of agents for calming, such as seizure disorder or sleep apnea, making a thorough history and accurate medication reconciliation essential. This complex medical presentation may suggest the need to modify ED general guidelines for patients with ASD. Both risperidone and olanzapine can be very useful when an antipsychotic effect and calming are needed. Risperidone is approved by the Food and Drug Administration for the treatment of severe irritability, aggression, and self-injurious behaviors in the pediatric population with autism[32,33] and is useful in nonemergency and emergency settings. Olanzapine has been less studied then risperidone, particularly in children, but is also recommended in general for emergency settings.[34] The oral dissolvable form of olanzapine may be especially helpful in pediatric patients with ASD with agitation, and an intramuscular formulation is also available. For patients with severe medical complications, midazolam, a short-acting benzodiazepine, can be beneficial as a first-line medication. It can be administered orally or nasally if intravenous therapy is not easily obtained.[33,35–38] In at least one case report, the oral combination of ketamine and midazolam has been used successfully in a combative patient with autism.[39] Olanzapine was studied under placebo control[40] in children with mental retardation and found to have a 50% response rate for the treatment of disruptive behaviors. Risperidone can safely be combined with a benzodiazepine, generally lorazepam in the case of pediatric patients.[34] With all psychotropic medications used in pediatric patients with ASD, the directive to start lower and go slower is a good guide, even in emergency situations. Hence, a recommendation is to start with lowered doses in the range of olanzapine 2.5 to 5.0 mg, risperidone 0.5 to 1.0 mg, and lorazepam 0.5 to 1.0 mg. It is important to point out that no studies of dosage in emergency settings involving children are noted in the literature. Lorazepam is used with caution because of the possibility of disinhibition and "could send the child over the edge,"[41] especially in the pediatric population with ASD.

MANAGEMENT OF PATIENTS WITH ACUTE AGITATION

The suggested ED least-restrictive treatment model for ASD with acute agitation can be seen in **Fig. 1**.

Rapid Assessment of Acute Agitation

The initial step is to complete a brief medical/nursing assessment. The ED practitioner should include the parent/caregiver in the evaluation process. Allowing the family member to ask the questions involved in the evaluation process can increase the likelihood of getting more accurate information on the suspected cause for the presenting concerns.

Adapting the care and treatment around the core features of ASD can significantly reduce agitation and improve positive treatment outcomes in acute care settings.[3] The physician/practitioner should quickly attempt to assess the patients' ability to follow directives and assess the level of cognitive abilities and input mode (visual, auditory, tactile) and the speed of processing (ie, single vs multistep directives).

Environmental Adaptations (Stimulation, Lighting, Number of People)

If at all possible, patients with ASD should be directed to a quiet room or area of the ED with minimal stimuli. Lighting should be lowered and noise levels should be reduced[42]; pagers, phones, and intercoms should be turned off. The number of staff used to care for patients should be kept to a minimum. Move slowly and explain how and why you need to touch patients during an examination or treatment, especially when you are about to touch them with medical equipment. Metal, plastic, or other objects of different temperatures can produce an atypical reaction. Other ED equipment, such

Complete brief Functional Behavior Assessment/Nursing- Medical Assessment

Adapt the ED environment including physical space, low lighting/
stimulation, include caregivers/family/support staff increase ER staff

Communication Adaptations (Non-verbal and verbal)- Linear/
Sequential/First Then/Modeling/Demonstration

Counseling/Contingency Management
CBT-Incentives/rewards – primary and secondary (stickers, tokens, edibles)

Relaxation Training – (sensory interventions) possibly offer PRN medications

Physically direct patient to a less stimulating and calming area

Blocking techniques – cushions/Pads – in lieu of hands on/restraints

Safety plan – unresponsive to lesser restrictive approaches – imminent risk/
danger - Restraints/Seclusion

Fig. 1. Least-restrictive treatment model for ASD in EDs. CBT, cognitive behavior therapy; ER, emergency room; PRN, Pro Re Nata.

as adhesive tape, creams, or patches, can also be difficult for patients with ASD who are tactile defensive.[43] Using verbal or visual demonstrations with a clear explanation of what you plan to do in advance is also helpful in reducing anxiety. Depending on the ability of the patients and the situation, also consider presenting a brief Social Story™ (the Gray Center, Grandville, MI) to patients explaining the procedures.

Communication
Communication is a critical area for all patients receiving treatment in emergency situations. Verbal and nonverbal communication adaptations (pictorial, Social Stories™, schedules, Picture Exchange, and picture schedules, and augmentative communication systems [talkers; iPad, Apple Inc, Cupertino, CA]) have been documented as effective ways to communicate with individuals with ASD.[44–46] Being aware of body language and nonverbal signs can help divert meltdowns, tantrums, and escalating behaviors related to frustration, lack of control/self-determination, and sensory overload.[47,48] Individuals may have fleeting eye contact or avoid it altogether. During periods of acute agitation, individuals on the autism spectrum may seem deaf and not respond to directives and may not be able to express wants, needs, or feelings, including

pain. When giving directives, present requests in a linear, sequential fashion (first open your mouth, then say ah). Stay away from using metaphors and synonyms or making analogies. As a result of a potential lag in response, give plenty of time for patients to respond to questions. It is important in many instances to repeat the questions or directives so that patients clearly understand the expectations. Be aware that some individuals with autism will say what you want them to say and not necessarily what they mean.

Behavioral approaches
Attempt to gain information on behavioral approaches that may be effective in reducing agitation of patients at home, school, or in the community. Applied behavior analysis and cognitive behavior therapy approaches that use incentives/rewards are considered evidence based and best practice for children on the autism spectrum. EDs should have access to a variety of possible incentives, such as candy, pretzels, pudding, stickers, cards, books, crayons, markers, tokens, videos, and cause-and-effect toys that make sounds or light up.

Somatosensory interventions
Somatosensory interventions can also be effective nonpharmacologic methods to treat acute agitation. Relaxation using sensory intervention techniques has been effective for reducing anxiety, aggression, and self-injury in some children with ASD. Some children and adults with autism may display atypical and paradoxic responses to sensory stimuli, specifically both over-reactivity and under-reactivity. Interventions in all sensory domains should be considered, including auditory (music, head phones); visual (photos, books, videos); tactile (brushing, deep pressure, weighted vests/blankets, heat wraps, cold, massage/touch); olfactory (scratch-and-sniff stickers, markers, flavored lip balm); and vestibular physical exercise or movement activity (swings). (Rocking chairs have been reported in the literature to reduce anxiety.) The caregivers of patients should be queried on the effective techniques because individual responses may vary.[47–49]

Restraint and Seclusion for Agitated Patients with ASD in the ED

In extremely agitated patients whereby the behavior exhibited interferes with the health, safety, and welfare of the patients or staff, restraint or seclusion may be necessary. State and national regulators have recognized the risks inherent in using any type of restraint (physical, mechanical, or chemical) and have set standards on provision of care that should be learned and followed by each practitioner.[50] Definitions of restraint include the following: any manual method, physical or mechanical device, material, or equipment that immobilizes or reduces the ability of a patient to move his or her arms, legs, body, or head freely or a drug or medication that is used as a restriction to manage the patient's behavior or restrict the patient's freedom of movement and not as a standard treatment or dosage for the patient's condition. Restraints do not include devices, such as orthopedically prescribed devices, surgical dressings or bandages, protective helmets, or other methods, that involve the physical holding of a patient for the purpose of conducting routine physical examinations or tests. Seclusion is the involuntary confinement of a patient alone in a room or area from which the patient is physically prevented from leaving.[50] Seclusion may be used only for safety and the management of violent or destructive behavior.

Caution When Using Restraint and Seclusion in Patients with ASD

Restraint and seclusion should not be used as punishment, to coerce or inflict pain, used in lieu of adequate staffing patterns, for staff convenience, or used simultaneously with seclusion (a patient alone in restraint behind a locked door). When it is determined that a patient's behavior is presenting as an imminent risk or danger to self and/or others or the person's behavior is interfering with life-sustaining treatment, the use of restraints may be indicated. The initial step is to determine the reason for restraint (medical/nonviolent or behavioral/psychiatric). Special devices made to reduce the chance of injury during physical restraint, such as vests or boards, should be used rather than sheets or clothing to restrain patients. Restraints should only be used as a last resort and only for the amount of time needed to complete a medical procedure or reduce the risk/danger that will alleviate the acute agitation or crisis situation. A risk assessment should also be obtained before using restraints or seclusion. The risk-assessment information may suggest modifications, adaptations, or refraining from using these interventions. Precautions may include advance directives (medical and behavioral health); pregnancy; heart and asthma conditions; history of fracture; seizure disorder; obesity; profile for excited delirium; head and spinal cord injury; and history of trauma or abuse (physical/sexual/emotional). The least-restrictive treatment option is defined as that treatment that affords the most favorable risk-to-benefit ratio, with specific consideration of the probability of treatment success, anticipated duration of treatment, distress caused by procedures, and distress caused by the behavior itself.

DISCUSSION

There is a paucity of literature on the best approach for providing treatment to children, adolescents, and adults with ASD presenting with acute agitation to the ED. A recent study found in a population-based data set that ED visits among youth with ASD were far more likely to be for psychiatric reasons when compared with visits among children without ASD.[51] Vulnerability of individuals on the autism spectrum regardless of their ability level includes reduced capacity to withstand stress, difficulty in expressing wants and needs, poor coping and problem solving skills, emotional lability, and executive-functioning deficits (speed of processing and problem solving). ED clinical staff currently receive minimal formal training and have limited experience with treating children, adolescents, and adults with ASD. As a result of their limited training, individuals with ASD have difficulty in receiving timely and appropriate medical care.[2,3,36] With the prevalence of autism on the rise and the increase of underdiagnosed and undiagnosed adults with ASD with comorbid medical and behavioral health needs, the need for prehospital and ED practitioners to have an understanding of ASD is critical in the diagnosis and treatment of medical and behavioral health conditions in acute care and crisis settings. With increased training and research and improvement in diagnostic tools, medical and behavioral health care personnel can improve the accuracy of diagnosing the underlying cause for acute agitation, provide effective treatment and interventions, and reduce unwanted treatment outcomes for individuals with ASD in acute care settings. A primary goal of health care providers in acute care settings should be to provide safe and effective care while improving the efficacy of the treatment outcomes using a least-restrictive/intrusive treatment model that, in turn, will improve the satisfaction of patients, families, and staff.

SUMMARY

There continues to be a paucity of literature regarding the treatment of patients with ASD in acute care and ED settings. Staff training efforts for ED personnel should draw on theories in nursing, child development, pain management, psychology, psychiatry, and applied behavior analysis.[52] Every person with ASD is unique, and treatment and interventions need to be individualized to patients and their families during emergency treatment and in the crisis situation. Adapting existing medical and behavioral health protocols in the ED to meet the needs of patients with ASD and their families will ultimately lead to more successful outcomes.

REFERENCES

1. Bradley E, Lofchy J. Learning disability in the accident and emergency department. Adv Psychiatr Treat 2005;11:345–57.
2. Smith MD, Graveline PJ, Smith JB. Autism and obstacles to medical diagnosis and treatment: two case studies. Focus on Autism and other Developmental Disabilities 2012;27(3):189–95.
3. Scarpinato N, Bradley J, Kurbjun K, et al. Caring for the child with an autism spectrum disorder in the acute care setting. J Spec Pediatr Nurs 2010;15(3): 244–54.
4. Unwanted outcomes – police contact & urgent hospital care. Bureau of Autism Services, Pennsylvania Department of Public Welfare. Pennsylvania autism needs assessment: a survey of individuals and families living with autism: unwanted outcomes-police contact & urgent hospital care. 2011. Available at: http://www.paautism.org/asert/Needs%20Assess_UnwantedOutcomes_Sept%202011.pdf. Accessed January 14, 2013.
5. American Psychiatric Association. Diagnostic and statistical manual of mental disorders, text revision (DSM IV - TR), vol. IV. Washington, DC: American Psychiatric Association; 2000.
6. Gabriels RL, Hill DE. Growing up with autism: working with school-age children and adolescents. New York: Guilford; 2007.
7. Gabriels RL. Adolescent transition to adulthood and vocational issues. In: Amaral D, Dawson G, Geschwind D, editors. Autism spectrum disorders. New York: Oxford University Press; 2011. p. 1167–81.
8. Gabriels RL, Cuccaro ML, Hill DE, et al. Repetitive behaviors in autism: relationships with associated clinical features. Res Dev Disabil 2005;26(2): 169–81.
9. Leekam SR, Nieto C, Libby SJ, et al. Describing the sensory abnormalities in children and adults with autism. J Autism Dev Disord 2007;37:894–910.
10. Leyfer OT, Folstein SE, Bacalman S. Comorbid psychiatric disorders in children with autism: interview development and rates of disorders. J Autism Dev Disord 2006;36:849–61.
11. Tuchman R, Rapin I. Epilepsy in autism. Lancet Neurol 2002;1(6):352–8.
12. Gabriels RL, Agnew JA, Miller LJ, et al. Is there a relationship between restricted, repetitive, stereotyped behaviors and interests and abnormal sensory response in children with autism spectrum disorders. Research Autism Spectrum Disorders 2008;2:660–70.
13. Baranek GT, David FJ, Poe MD, et al. Sensory experiences questionnaire: discriminating sensory features in young children with autism, developmental delays, and typical development. J Child Psychol Psychiatry 2006;47(6):591–601.
14. Tecchio T, Benassi F, Zappasodi F, et al. Auditory sensory processing in autism: a magnetoencephalographic study. Biol Psychiatry 2003;54:647–54.
15. Tomchek SD, Dunn W. Sensory processing in children with and without autism: a comparative study using the short sensory profile. Am J Occup Ther 2007;61(2): 190–200.
16. Centers for Disease Control and Prevention. Autism spectrum disorder data & statistics. 2010. Available at: http://www.cdc.gov/ncbddd/autism/data.html. Accessed December 21, 2011.

17. Mandell DS, Thompson WW, Weintraub ES, et al. Trends in diagnosis rates for autism and ADHD at hospital discharge in the context of other psychiatric diagnoses. Psychiatr Serv 2005;56(1):56–62.
18. Simonoff E, Pickles A, Charman T, et al. Psychiatric disorders in children with autism spectrum disorders: prevalence, comorbidity, and associated factors in a population-derived sample. J Am Acad Child Adolesc Psychiatry 2008;8:921–9.
19. Eldridge C, Kennedy R. Nonpharmacologic techniques for distress reduction during emergency medical care: a review. Clin Pediatr Emerg Med 2010; 11(4):244–50.
20. Volkmar FR, Nelson DS. Seizures disorders in autism. J Am Acad Child Adolesc Psychiatry 1990;29(1):127–9.
21. Schreck KA, Mulick JA, Smith AF. Sleep problems as possible predictors of intensified symptoms of autism. Res Dev Disabil 2004;25:57–66.
22. Gabriels R, Beresford C. Outcomes of a short-term specialized intensive care psychiatric hospital program for pediatric patients with autism spectrum disorders. Abstract presented at the 59th Annual Meeting of the American Academy of Child and Adolescent Psychiatry. San Francisco, CA, October 25, 2012.
23. LeCavalier L. Behavioral and emotional problems in young people with pervasive developmental disorders: relative prevalence, effects of subject characteristics, and empirical classification. J Autism Dev Disord 2006;36:1101–14.
24. Ghaziuddin M. Asperger syndrome: associated psychiatric and medical conditions. Focus Autism Other Dev Disabl 2002;27(3):138–44.
25. Dorland's medical dictionary for health consumers. Philadelphia, PA: Saunders; 2007.
26. Nordstrom K, Zun LS, Wilson MP. Medical evaluation and triage of the agitated patient: consensus statement of the American Association for Emergency Psychiatry Project Beta Medical Evaluation Workgroup. West J Emerg Med 2012; 13(1):3–10.
27. Venkat A, Jauch E, Russell WS. Care of the patient with an autism spectrum disorder by the general physician. Postgrad Med J 2012;88(1042):472–81.
28. Miano S, Ferri R. Epidemiology and management of insomnia in children with autistic spectrum disorders. Paediatr Drugs 2010;12:75–84.
29. Richmond JS, Berlin JS, Fishkind AB, et al. Verbal de-escalation of the agitated patient: consensus statement of the American Association for Emergency Psychiatry Project Beta De-escalation Workgroup. West J Emerg Med 2011;13: 17–25.
30. Knox DK, Holloman GH. Use and avoidance of seclusion and restraint: consensus statement of the American Association for Emergency Psychiatry Project Beta Seclusion and Restraint Workgroup. West J Emerg Med 2012;13: 35–40.
31. Owley TB. Treatment with individuals with autism spectrum disorders in emergency department: special considerations. Clin Pediatr Emerg Med 2004;5: 187–92.
32. McCracken J, McGough J, Shah B. Risperidone in children with autism and serious behavioural problems. N Engl J Med 2002;347:314–21.
33. Aman MG, Crismon ML, Frances A, et al. Treatment of psychiatric and behavior problems in individuals with mental retardation: an update of the expert consensus guidelines for mental retardation/developmental disability population. Englewood (CO): Postgraduate Institute for Medicine; 2004.
34. Allen MH, Currier GW, Carpenter D, et al. Treatment of behavioral emergencies. J Psychiatr Pract 2005;11(Suppl 1):4–112.

35. Lane RD, Schunk JE. Atomized intranasal midazolam use for minor procedures in the pediatric emergency department. Pediatr Emerg Care 2008;24:300–3.
36. Ljungman G, Kreuger A, Andreasson S, et al. Midazolam nasal spray reduces procedural anxiety in children. Pediatrics 2000;105:73–8.
37. Pisalchalyong T, Trairatuorakul C, Jirakijja J, et al. Comparison of the effectiveness of oral diazepam and midazolam for the sedation of autistic patients during dental treatment. Pediatr Dent 2005;27:198–206.
38. Fukuta O, Braqham RL, Yanase H, et al. The sedative effect of intranasal midazolam administration in the dental treatment of patients with mental disabilities. J Clin Pediatr Dent 1993;17:231–7.
39. Shah S, Shah S, Apuya J, et al. Combination of oral ketamine and midazolam as a premedication for a severely autistic and combative patient. J Anesth 2009;23:126–8.
40. Hollander E, Wasserman S, Swanson EN, et al. A double-blind placebo-controlled pilot study of olanzapine in childhood-adolescent pervasive developmental disorder. J Child Adolesc Psychopharmacol 2006;16:541–8.
41. Chun T. Autism demands attention in the emergency room. ACEP news; 2012. Available at: http://www.acepnews.com/index.php?id=495. Accessed January 13, 2013.
42. Sullivan MG. Autism demands attention in the emergency department. ACEP News; 2012. Available at: www.acepnews.com/index.php?id=514&;txttnews%5Bttnews%5D=1255&cHash=55a3d518ca585feef2b99fb978fbf035. Accessed January 4, 2013.
43. Autism Society of America (ASA). Tips for first responders. Available at: http://www.autism-society.org/living-with-autism/how-we-can-help/safe-and-sound/tips-for-first-responders.html. Accessed January 8, 2013.
44. Bondy AS, Frost LA. The picture exchange communication system. Focus Autistic Behavior 1994;9(3):1–19.
45. Scattone D, Wilczynski SM, Edwards RP, et al. Decreasing disruptive behaviors of children with autism using social stories. J Autism Dev Disord 2002;32:535–43.
46. Crozier S, Tincani MJ. Using a modified social story TM to decrease disruptive behavior of a child with autism. Focus Autism Other Dev Disabl 2005;20:150–7.
47. Notbohm E. Ten things every child with autism wishes you knew, updated and expanded edition. Future Herizon; 2012. Available at: www.ellennotbohm.com/article-archive/ten-things-every-child-with-autism-wishes. Accessed January 15, 2013.
48. Finke EH, Light J, Kitko L. A systematic review of the effectiveness of nurse communication with patients with complex communication needs with a focus on the use of augmentative and alternative communication. J Clin Nurs 2008;17:2102–15.
49. Hodgetts S, Hodgetts W. Somatosensory stimulation interventions for children with autism: literature review and clinical considerations. Can J Occup Ther 2007;74(5):393–400.
50. Joint Commission, CMS on Provision of Care. The Joint Commission, comprehensive accreditation manual for behavioral health, 2009, PC-53.
51. Kalb LG, Sturat EA, Freeman B, et al. Psychiatric-related emergency departments visits among children with autism spectrum disorders. Pediatr Emerg Care 2012;28(12):1269–76.
52. Sounders MC, Freeman KG, DePaul D, et al. Caring for children and adolescents with autism who require challenging procedures. Pediatr Nurs 2002;28(6):555–62.

Systems of Care for Individuals with Autism Spectrum Disorder and Serious Behavioral Disturbance Through the Lifespan

Martin J. Lubetsky, MD[a],*, Benjamin L. Handen, PhD, BCBA-D[a],
Michelle Lubetsky, MEd, BCBA[b], John J. McGonigle, PhD[a]

KEYWORDS

- Autism • Systems of care • Service delivery • Early intervention
- Department of Developmental and Intellectual Disabilities • Department of Education
- Department of Mental Health/Behavioral Health • Office of Vocational Rehabilitation

KEY POINTS

- Parents request guidance and instruction from professionals after the diagnosis of Autism Spectrum Disorder/Intellectual Disability is confirmed because many complex systems are involved.
- The education system is directed by the Individuals with Disabilities Education Act, including the Individual Education Plan, which must be tailored to fit the needs of the child and adolescent.
- The Intellectual Disability system has supports to assist with the pursuit of waiver funding and individualized services, and to prepare and monitor the Individual Support Plan.
- The Mental Health/Behavioral Health System offers service coordinators to assist with finding resources and individualized services.
- The Medical System is complex and requires providers who are knowledgeable and able to coordinate primary care, dental, vision, nutrition, and other specialists to promote integration into a "medical home model of care."

INTRODUCTION

Individuals with Autism Spectrum Disorder (ASD) have unique needs, and interventions must be individualized for successful outcomes. It is beneficial to optimize

Disclosure Statement: None (M.J. Lubetsky, J.J. McGonigle, M. Lubetsky); B.L. Handen has received industry research support from Eli Lilly, Bristol Myers Squibb, and Curemark. He also has received research support from Autism Speaks, HRSA, NIA, and NIMH.
[a] Department of Psychiatry, Western Psychiatric Institute and Clinic of UPMC, University of Pittsburgh School of Medicine, 3811 O'Hara Street, Pittsburgh, PA 15213, USA; [b] Allegheny Intermediate Unit, 475 Waterfront Drive East, Homestead, PA 15120, USA
* Corresponding author.
E-mail address: lubetskymj@upmc.edu

coordination of care, similar to the "medical home" model, for the primary care physician. Many systems may be involved to provide services or funding resources and support to assist persons with ASD and/or Intellectual Disability (ID) and their families. More systems and services are available for children and adolescents with ASD/ID than for adults. Therefore, when adolescents leave the education system, they face greater challenges in obtaining services. There are also many hurdles during transitions from pediatric primary care and child behavioral health services to vocational services, adult medical care, and adult behavioral health services. Lubetsky and coworkers[1] have provided a comprehensive description of levels of care and services across the lifespan and a detailed list of references.

Coordination of multiple services is a challenge for families. For example, in the state of Pennsylvania, child systems include the following: Child Find, Alliance for Infants and Toddlers, early intervention services, local education systems, pediatrics, the Department of Developmental or Intellectual Disability/Autism, and the Department of Mental Health/Behavioral Health. At times, Child Protection Services/Child Welfare and Juvenile Detention may also be involved.

Adult systems in the state include the Department of Developmental or Intellectual Disability/Autism, the Department of Mental Health/Behavioral Health, and the Office of Vocational Rehabilitation. Other systems, such as junior colleges or universities, employers, and housing agencies, may also have important roles to play.

SYSTEMS OF CARE IN ASD ACROSS THE COUNTRY

States throughout the country are monitoring the increased prevalence of ASD and the growing numbers of adolescents transitioning to adulthood.[2] Most states are attempting to develop systems of care to meet the needs of individuals from early childhood through adulthood and their families.[3] However, the ever-changing economic climate impacts funding streams for ASD/ID services under federal, state, and county line items, as well as Medicaid, Medicare, and private insurance.[4]

Many states strive to develop systems of care that include screening, diagnostic assessment, information and referrals, early intervention, behavioral support, applied behavioral analysis/functional behavior assessment, in-home care, skill training, parent training and education, respite care, case management, service coordination, supportive housing, supported employment, self-directed services—person-centered planning processes, service care planning, individualized budgeting, and quality assurance. In an effort to identify best treatment practices across the country, the National Standards Project reviewed intervention models and provided a best practices list of recommended services for children with ASD.[5]

The Center for System Change reviewed several state reports, and although recommendations cover many issues that impact individuals with ASD, there were several gaps identified.[6] For example, Iowa identified the needs of siblings of individuals with ASD and recommended increased awareness and training. Cultural diversity is another area highlighted for better sensitivity and training. In addition, the report noted that although the need for mental health/behavioral health services is great, only 2 in 5 children with disabilities and poor psycho-social adjustment receive mental health services. Schools were identified as a critical site for behavioral health support, as well as the development of models for social skills training for students with ASD.

Much effort has focused on training pediatricians in identification of early warning signs of ASD and development of an autism pediatric practice "medical home" model.[7,8] The "medical home" is designed to provide coordinated, accessible, continuous, culturally competent care, screening, education, referrals, and follow-up.[9,10] The University of Wisconsin Waisman Center has developed a Primary Care model for training pediatricians and family practitioners in ASD.[11] The Help Autism Now Society has developed an Autism Physician Handbook with curriculum, scripts, and a DVD.[12] With the growing number of adolescents transitioning into adulthood, there is increased need for a similar adult "medical home" model and associated training materials.[13]

There is often uncertainty concerning where to refer and who will assist the child and family. As a result, emergency department visits among children with ASD and challenging behaviors has increased. A recent survey by Kalb and coworkers[14] found that 13% of visits among children with ASD were due to psychiatric/behavioral problems compared with 2% of all visits by youth without ASD. The study's conclusion was that there is great need for improving community-based psychiatric/behavioral health systems of care for youth with ASD to divert emergency department visits for psychiatric-related reasons.

Several individual state reports have provided important findings. The Department of Public Welfare in Pennsylvania convened the Autism Task Force and published a final report in 2004 resulting in the establishment of the Bureau of Autism Services (BAS) within the Office of Developmental Programs.[15] The PA Autism Needs Assessment was developed by the BAS, who published the final report in 2011.[16] They found that needs existed in the range of services, barriers, and limitations to accessing services, obtaining a diagnosis and follow-up care, family impact, employment challenges, and finding crisis response services for challenging behaviors. As a result of this needs assessment, 3 regional autism centers in western, central, and eastern parts of the state were established with a partnership between universities, the state, and local agencies and families. These centers spearheaded the training of pediatric offices in early warning signs and referral for diagnostic assessment of ASD. In addition, an adult autism waiver was initiated to fund services for selected individuals older than age 21 without other state waiver funding (such as ID). The BAS promotes innovation and evidence-based services, fills gaps in care, and strives for advocacy and policy change. They work with early intervention, Behavioral Health and Rehabilitation Services, Department of Education, Office of Developmental Programs (which offers ID waivers), and Medicaid program Healthchoices (which covers managed care plans).

To be eligible for the Pennsylvania Adult Autism Waiver, a person must be age 21 or older, a United States citizen, and resident of Pennsylvania and meet certain diagnostic, financial, and functional eligibility criteria.[17] Priority is given to those not already receiving ongoing state funded or state and federally funded long-term care services. Eligibility criteria include the following: a diagnosis of an ASD; income and resource limits for Medicaid met; and substantial functional limitations existing that are likely to continue indefinitely in 3 or more of the major life activities (self-care, understanding and use of receptive and expressive language, learning, mobility, self-direction, capacity for independent living).

The Pennsylvania Adult Community Autism Program (ACAP) provides physical, behavioral, and community services to adults with ASD.[18] ACAP is specifically designed to help adults with ASD participate in their communities based on individual needs and interests. Eligibility criteria include 21 years of age or older; eligible for Medicaid; diagnosis of an ASD; certified as requiring services at the level of an Intermediate Care Facility; not enrolled in a Medicaid Home and Community Based Waiver program; able to live in a community without 16 or more awake paid and unpaid staff supervision hours per day without presenting a danger to self or others or a threat to property; 3 or more substantial functional limitations in the following areas of major life activity: self-care, receptive and expressive language, learning, mobility, self-direction, or capacity for independent living; not enrolled in a Medicaid-managed care organization; and not enrolled in the Health Insurance Premium Payment Program. ACAP is currently available in 4 Pennsylvania counties: Dauphin, Cumberland, Chester, and Lancaster. ACAP Services includes all physician services (including emergency services provided by a physician, psychiatric services, direct access to a woman's health specialist, and several other adjunct services).

California has a comprehensive developmental disabilities services program through mandated legislation, the Lanterman Act of 2010, that supports best practices for ASD screening, diagnostic assessment, and development of standards for effectiveness. A subsequent report identified areas of need: obtaining a diagnosis, quality-of-life issues, acceptance of ASD in the community, access to health care, systems of care, ease of navigating systems, treatment, service quality, health insurance, school districts, transitioning to adult services, higher education, employment, and residential services.[19]

Indiana developed the HANDS in Autism Interdisciplinary Training and Resource Center through the Christian Sarkine Autism Treatment Center at Riley Children's Hospital at Indiana University Health and the IU School of Medicine. Their goal is to develop a model system of training that will facilitate the development of local capacity within schools, service providers, and communities to serve individuals with ASD and their families. A Toolkit for Medical Professionals was developed to provide training for professionals with the goal of fostering collaboration across multiple systems and environments.[20]

Missouri developed their statewide Autism Centers of Excellence and funded 4 regional centers across the state. Their goals include the following: to reduce wait times from first symptoms to diagnosis, provide information, manage referrals, and train community-based service providers.[21]

Massachusetts reviewed the maze of services and developed their own autism waiver program. The Office of Medicaid and the Department of Developmental Services Autism Division offers an Autism Waiver Program for children age birth through 8. The Waiver allows children to receive expanded habilitation and education (in-home services and supports, such as Applied Behavioral Analysis for a total of 3 years).[22]

New Hampshire developed the "Building a Circle of Care" model to respond to a lack of coordination of care. The primary members include the following: medical home (primary care physician, dentist, specialist, insurance carrier), special education, therapeutic interventions (Behavior Analyst Certification Board, speech, occupational therapy, behavioral health, and insurance carrier), family support (family, parent-to-parent, respite), community support (service coordinator, support groups), and the individual with ASD in the middle of the circle. Their Web site lists "what to expect from..." each of the various types of providers.[23]

Maryland's recommendations for an autism statewide system of care included partnering with organizations and systems to establish regional collaborative hubs, as well as developing a "customized employment model" for adults.[24] The state of Washington's resource for individuals, families, and professionals assessed the full age spectrum and medical systems, including primary care, dental, nutrition, as well as psychiatric and behavioral issues.[25]

In addition, private insurance mandates have been legislated across many states to mandate coverage for ASD diagnosis and intervention.[26] As of August 2012, a total of 37 states and the District of Columbia had laws related to ASD and insurance coverage from comprehensive to limited coverage for children less than the age of 21 with ASD.[27] For example, in Pennsylvania, Act 62 was passed in 2008 to cover up to $36,000 in ASD-related diagnostic and treatment services.[28] The New York Health Plan Association report focused on managed care and how to manage ASD insurance mandates across several states.[29] The report highlights the need for every relationship to be built on physical, behavioral, and social care coordination and information sharing.

THE MENTAL HEALTH SYSTEM

Families often begin their first involvement with the mental health/behavioral health system after a child has been diagnosed with ASD. Children with ASD who experience significant behavioral challenges may be referred for treatment by psychologists, social workers, or behavioral specialists. In cases where medication for management of behavioral/emotional problems is indicated, a child psychiatrist or developmental pediatrician may be consulted. These providers may be working within a private practice, be affiliated with a mental health clinic, or work within a developmental or autism clinic at an outpatient hospital setting. In several states, intensive early intervention services, such as Applied Behavior Analysis or Floor Time, are also available through mental health agencies. These services are often provided in the home, consisting of 20 to 40 hours a week of individualized instruction.[30] Depending on the state, such services may be funded through mental health dollars, private insurance, education system, or out of pocket by the family. These services include early intensive intervention in home, in preschool, or in clinic, as well as parent psycho-education, support, and behavioral strategy training.

As the child gets older, there may be the need for services in outpatient, home, school, or inpatient/residential setting. The following list of services may apply for adolescents and adults as well:

- Outpatient individual, group, or family therapies
- In-home behavioral support and parent behavioral strategy training
- In-school behavioral support and teacher behavioral strategy training
- Intensive Outpatient Program consisting of group, individual, and family therapies and medication interventions
- Partial Hospital Program/Day Treatment, if behaviors are too severe to return to school, provides group, individual, family, and medication interventions
- Community or Mental Health Crisis Services provides crisis-trained staff to help an individual and family during a crisis when safety is at risk.
- Acute Psychiatric Hospital treatment provides crisis management, diagnostic and treatment services, stabilization of acute symptoms and plans for discharge and reintegration in a brief stay. If these school, community, in-home, intensive and acute psychiatric inpatient services are not successful, and the child can no longer function safely in the family or community setting, then a longer stay intensive treatment program is needed.
- Residential Treatment Facility or Intensive Treatment Unit may be necessary for longer stay than inpatient hospitalization. A Residential Treatment Facility provides intensive treatment and skills training focus with strong family involvement.

FAMILY SUPPORT SERVICES

Family support is available through several sources, depending on the locality. Many states offer some form of case management or services/supports coordination. For example, in Pennsylvania, families are able to register their child for a support coordinator under the Office of Developmental Programs if the child meets criteria for ID, to serve as an advocate and develop the Individual Support Plan. A services coordinator under Mental Health/Behavioral Health can be obtained through one of their local mental health clinics to assist the family in obtaining appropriate services for the child. These forms of case management also apply for adolescents and adults.

Respite care provides short-term, temporary living arrangements to families caring for an individual with disabilities and can occur in the home of the individual, at home, or at a facility. Sometimes the family has a need for a preplanned respite for their child to permit the family to take a vacation or when other family members are not able to provide support. Some states have an emergency respite model that is meant for an acute behavioral crisis and requires extra training and staffing. The need for respite may also apply for adolescents and adults.

Finally, there are several nationwide ASD advocacy groups that offer a wide range of supportive services to families. Autism Speaks and the Autism Society of America often have local chapters with staff that is able to assist families in finding resources and obtaining services. Autism Speaks has a "100 Day Kit" for families of children newly diagnosed with ASD (as well as a "100 Day Kit" for families of newly diagnosed children with Asperger disorder) and also offers several tool kits that are available to families on-line (covering topics such as sleep issues, toilet training, and visits to the dentist). Some local chapters conduct parent support groups and offer workshops on topics of importance to families, educators, and clinicians.

THE MEDICAL SYSTEM AND ALLIED HEALTH PROFESSIONALS

Once an ASD diagnosis has been determined, the medical system may also play an important role in addressing issues related to ASD. For example, many families are referred for genetic testing following an ASD diagnosis. As many children with ASD have other medical issues, specialists such as gastroenterologists, neurologists, or sleep specialists may also be consulted. Many families use the services of private speech and language therapists or occupational therapists, who are often affiliated with medical centers or, in some cases, may be in private practice.

The "Medical Home" integrated primary care pediatrics or adult medicine model describes that the primary care doctor manages the overall health care, provides referrals, and maintains communication with other health care providers, including physical health and behavioral health services. Referrals and collaboration can include speech/language therapy, occupational therapy, physical therapy, and nutrition/dietician.

ILLUSTRATIVE AUTISM PROGRAM EXAMPLE

The Center for Autism and Developmental Disorders at Western Psychiatric Institute and Clinic of UPMC (WPIC) and University of Pittsburgh School of Medicine serves children, adolescents and adults from a tri-state area (Pennsylvania, Ohio, West Virginia, as well as other states and countries). The Center's mission is to provide high-quality evidence-based clinical services in a seamless continuum of care, curriculum-based training of medical and other allied health students and professionals, and clinical research. The Center has services for children as young as 18 months of age through adults in their senior years. Most services are insurance-based, whether Medicaid, private insurance, or Medicare. There are many levels of care, including hospital acute care services, ambulatory/community programs, and support services.

Hospital Acute Care Services:

- *WPIC Psychiatric Diagnostic Evaluation/Emergency Center* provides 24-hour/ 7-day-a-week emergency assessment of any age individual with any diagnosis for acute behavioral symptoms.
- *WPIC Re:solve Crisis Intervention Services* include phone response, 2-person team mobile response, crisis center site with emergency management, crisis intervention, and overnight stay.
- *Merck Program Specialized Inpatient Unit* is an acute care psychiatric hospital program for children, adolescents, and adults with ASD/ID and comorbid mental health disorders. The unit has 32 beds divided into 3 wings for appropriate placement based on age, gender, developmental level, acuity, and potential for dangerous behavior. The team consists of 2 child and adolescent psychiatrists, one adult psychiatrist, a behavioral psychologist, a nurse clinical manager, behavioral specialists, special education teachers, vocational specialists, psychiatric nurses, psychiatric social workers, a physician assistant or nurse practitioner, creative and expressive arts therapists, and milieu therapists. Family practice physicians and nutritionists/dieticians serve as in-house consultants. Other medical referrals are made to the adult or children's hospitals. Family involvement and intervention are part of every individual's treatment. Interagency collaboration with outside agencies/systems is a vital link to the community for disposition planning and successful outcomes. Teaching behavioral strategies to families, caregivers, and agency staff is a component of every treatment plan.

Ambulatory Child/Adolescent Programs:

- *Merck Program Specialized Child and Adolescent Outpatient Clinic* provides diagnostic evaluations for ASD/ID or other psychiatric disorders, individual, group, and family therapies, behavioral strategies, social skills training, as well as medication assessment and management.
- *Autism Treatment Network*, supported by Autism Speaks, provides a comprehensive assessment including possible medical concerns, such as issues around sleep, gastrointestinal/constipation, dental, neurology/seizures, and genetics.
- *Autism Early Intensive Behavioral Intervention Program* uses evidence-based Applied Behavioral Analysis Discrete Trial Training methodology in the home or school for up to 30 hours per week. Most funding is provided through Medicaid, unless a private insurance company has approved coverage.
- *Autism Therapeutic Preschool* provides Early Intensive Behavioral Intervention using evidence-based Applied Behavioral Analysis Discrete Trial Training methodology, as well as social skills interventions and family-based strengths support 6 hours a day, 5 days a week. Most funding is through Medicaid, unless a private insurance company has approved coverage.
- *Specialized Therapeutic Classrooms* in a center-based special education school provide an intensive day treatment setting for children ages 5 to 21. The treatment team includes a special education teacher, paraprofessionals, behavioral health clinicians, social worker, psychiatric nurse, and child and adolescent psychiatrist. Funding for the behavioral health team is through Medicaid.
- *Specialized Summer Intensive Day Treatment Program* provides a therapeutic setting to continue behavioral health treatment for 8 weeks, 5 days per week, 6 hours per day. The treatment team includes behavioral health clinicians, social

worker, psychiatric nurse, and child and adolescent psychiatrist. Funding is through Medicaid, private insurance, or an IEP-approved Extended School Year contract (if the school district has approved funding).

- *Specialized Summer Therapeutic Inclusion Program* allows children with ASD to attend a community day camp with therapeutic support for 8 weeks, 5 days per week, 6 hours per day. Parents pay tuition for camp, whereas the behavioral health clinicians are funded through Medicaid or private insurance company.
- *School consultation* may be provided to schools through individual contracts.
- *Specialized Family-based Mental Health* team provides intensive family support, intervention, case management, and crisis response for a prescribed period of time. Funding is through Medicaid.
- *Specialized Group Home Residential Mobile Treatment Team* works with group homes, which are funded through ID waiver funds, Behavioral Health funds, or Child Welfare System funds. The Mobile Treatment Team consists of a psychologist, behavioral specialist, family therapist, psychiatric social worker, psychiatric nurse, and child and adolescent psychiatrist funded through a Medicaid Behavioral Health carved out in Allegheny County for the most complex children and adolescents.

Ambulatory Adult Programs:

- *Merck Program Specialized Adult Outpatient Clinic* provides diagnostic evaluations for ASD/ID or other psychiatric disorders, individual, group, and family therapies, behavioral strategies, social skills training, medication assessment, and management.
- *Vocational Training Center* provides work skills training, independence training, structured day programming, and social support for adults with ID and is funded through ID waiver funds.
- *Supported Employment Program* provides job assessment, interview skills training, employer matching, and job coaching for adults with ASD/ID and is funded through ID waiver funds or the Office of Vocational Rehabilitation (if the adult does not have ID).

Support Services:

- *WPIC Telepsychiatry service* works with several county community mental health agencies that have a physician/nurse clinician team at their site. Also, there is a telepsychiatry pilot project that includes teachers in the medication appointments for their students who are seen in the clinic.
- *WPIC Service Coordinators* offer care coordination of mental health/behavioral health services.
- *Western Pennsylvania Regional Autism Center ASERT* (Autism Services Education Resources and Training) is funded by the state Department of Public Welfare Office of Developmental Programs Bureau of Autism Services. The Centers offer trainings, networking, resource referrals, pilot intervention projects, and expansion of services for adults.
- *Behavior Analysis Certification Program* (*approved by the international BACB board*) was developed by WPIC/UPMC and University of Pittsburgh Department of Special Education, which has increased the number of board-certified behavior specialists in autism in the region.
- *Community collaborations* are a component of the systems of care and there are many local parent support organizations and peer support programs.

EARLY CHILDHOOD SERVICE SYSTEMS

From the moment a young child receives a diagnosis of ASD, the child and his/her family will begin to develop important relationships with several service providers. Although the specific names of providers and systems may vary from state to state, the goals will be quite similar.

All states provide early intervention (EI) services to children with ASD.[31] Typically, EI services are provided in the home for infants and toddlers (until age 3) and in classrooms/preschools for children between the ages of 3 and 5 years. However, EI services in many states do not generally cover the intensity of services that is being recommended for young children with ASD. Some states may pay for these services through mental/behavioral health reimbursement, public and private insurance plans, or out of pocket by parents. Children are often identified as requiring EI services by the child's pediatrician or day-care staff. Following an assessment, specific services are recommended to address deficit areas. Ancillary services, such as speech and language therapy or occupational therapy, may be offered in private offices or specialized preschool programs. At certain milestones (eg, school entry), some providers will no longer be available as the child becomes eligible for different services.

THE EDUCATION SYSTEM

Services for school-age students with an ASD/ID diagnosis are guided by the Individuals with Disabilities Education Act (IDEA).[32] The law explains the educational rights of students with disabilities and describes eligibility requirements for children to receive special education supports and services.[33–35]

Entitlement is based on a 2-pronged requirement to determine if a child can receive special education services. First, the child must have one (or more) of the specific disabilities identified in IDEA. Second, the child must, as a result of that disability, demonstrate a need for specially designed instruction.

Legal protections are available for students under IDEA, and the following components of IDEA represent significant protections for students with disabilities. The Free and Appropriate Public Education states that it is every child's right, including those with disabilities, to receive a free and appropriate public education. In some cases, the term "appropriate" can lead to different interpretations. The Least Restrictive Environment states that children are to be educated in a setting with children without disabilities, to the maximum extent possible. The provision requires that the IEP team address individual educational placement decisions. The Individual Education Plan (IEP) is the legal document that is designed to represent individualized instructional programming for the student. It should be reviewed annually and modified, as needed, to promote progress toward goals. The IEP directs the educational program by addressing meaningful individual goals. Every child who receives special education services must have an IEP.

Students with ASD can be included in regular education, and the Least Restrictive Environment requires that the general education classroom be considered when placement decisions are made. All students must have access to the general education curriculum, to the extent appropriate. The team should determine if the addition of supplementary aids and services could allow the student to meet IEP goals within the general education setting. If the student requires supports and services that cannot be delivered in the general education classroom, then other options, such as receiving instruction outside of the regular classroom, may be considered.

Support services are available in schools for students with ASD, as described in IDEA, "Supplementary Aids and Services means aids, services, and other supports that are provided in regular education classes, other education-related settings, and in extracurricular and non-academic settings, to enable children with disabilities to be educated with nondisabled children to the maximum extent appropriate..." (IDEA 300.114-300.116). Aids and Services include specially designed instruction, such as accommodations and modifications to instruction. They can also include the manner in which content is presented, how a child's progress is measured, direct supports to the child, and support and training for staff who work with the child. Often, children with ASD benefit from additional itinerant services, such as speech and language therapy, occupational therapy, and counseling. Types of services are individually determined from evaluation data. In some situations, students with high functioning autism receive support without having an IEP. These students may be supported by school counselors and/or speech and language clinicians for social skill instruction.

If an IEP team determines that general classroom management techniques are insufficient to ameliorate challenging behavior and a student's behavior is interfering with his/her learning or the learning of others, then the IEP team should consider implementing a functional behavior assessment to guide the development of a positive behavior support plan. A positive behavior support plan should include methods that use positive behavioral techniques to shape a child's behavior. Using information derived from the functional behavior assessment, the least intrusive interventions should be selected for inclusion in the plan. The positive behavior support plan should be included in the IEP and everyone involved should be familiar with the implementation strategies to promote successful outcomes (IDEA 300.324(2)(i)).

If a comprehensive evaluation concludes that the student does not meet the 2-pronged criteria for special education then the Rehabilitation Act of 1973 may be relevant. The Act protects the rights of qualified individuals by prohibiting discrimination based on their disability. Section 504 of the Rehabilitation Act states that organizations that receive federal funds are required to make their programs accessible by providing reasonable accommodations to individuals with disabilities. Students with disabilities who do not qualify for the protections of IDEA may benefit from the development of a 504 plan with the school's 504 coordinator, committee, or team. The 504 plan document delineates specific accommodations that will be implemented by the school. All staff should be made aware of the accommodations and the plan should be reviewed annually. After implementing an initial 504 plan, a meeting should be scheduled within 6 weeks to review progress. Issuing a 504 plan does not provide the same level of protections as found in an IEP, but it can inform teachers of specific areas of need and direct them to implement accommodations that promote equal access to the curriculum.[36]

TRANSITION SERVICES TO ADULT SYSTEMS

By the time students with disabilities reach 16 years of age, the IEP must include documentation that reflects planning for services in postsecondary education/training, employment, and independent living goals. These efforts can help to prepare students to leave the entitlements afforded through IDEA and face the challenges of navigating the adult world. Access to adult systems is based on eligibility and fewer supports are available. During the transition from adolescence to adulthood, there is an even greater need for care coordination and collaborative care between systems; however, there is often a lack of providers who are knowledgeable and experienced in working with individuals with ASD/ID.

Adults with ASD/ID may need other supportive services that can impact challenging behaviors by providing structure and direction. If the individual with ASD has ID, then Community-Based Day Services/Adult Training Facilities are designed to provide specialized activities intended to structure a schedule of activities to enhance skill development and independent living. The supports are driven by individual need and are focused on increased functional independence, vocational training, and recreational activities. Supported Employment is another structured program designed to empower people by helping them find jobs within the community while receiving support from training specialists/job coaches. Training specialists/job coaches work with employers to prepare employees in a specific job. An in-depth job analysis is conducted and the employee is trained to carry out all tasks involved with that job. These services may include vocational evaluation, job search, help with application and interviews, building work relationships, community inclusive activities, and opportunities for community service.[37]

Several levels of mental health/behavioral health care exist for adults with ASD/ID and challenging behaviors, similar to services for children and adolescents, but more limited in availability. They range from outpatient diagnosis and treatment to crisis intervention and stabilization to acute psychiatric hospitalization. Often these services are provided in general psychiatric settings rather than in specialized programs. These options vary across states and insurance plans. A level of care that provides an alternative to acute psychiatric hospitalization for patients not needing 24-hour supervision is an acute or day partial hospital program. This service provides a high degree of therapeutic support, to develop effective coping and interpersonal skills, stress management, medication assessment, and reintegration into the community. If extended 24-hour mental health care is needed, a long-term structured residence is a highly structured mental health residential treatment facility that provides behavioral health treatment and specialized programming in a controlled environment with a high degree of supervision.

HOUSING OPTIONS

Many individuals with ASD/ID live at home with their families or with in-home supports; however, an increasing number of young adults seek alternative housing arrangements with limited options and inadequate funding. If the individual with ASD/ID has challenging behaviors that require out-of-home placement, there is a wide variety of options across states. One example of a mental health residential program is the Community Residential Rehabilitation Service, which is specifically designed to assist persons with chronic psychiatric disability to live as independently as possible through the provision of training and assistance in the skills of community living. The Community Residential Rehabilitation Service also serves as an integrating focus for the person's rehabilitation. An example of more restrictive residential settings for individuals with ID is the Intermediate Care Facilities for Developmental Disabilities, which are state or privately operated residential programs specifically designed to furnish health and rehabilitative services. Supervised group home living is another alternative that provides around-the-clock trained staff to support individuals on-site.

If the individual with ASD/ID desires to move to a more independent living setting, there are a range of options that differ across states. One alternative is Lifesharing (Family Living), which supports individuals with ID to live with qualified unrelated adults who provide support in their home. Another supported housing arrangement is supervised apartment living with staff to provide direction and emergency response. A more independent option is supported living, in which agency staff provide support several times a week to teach budgeting, purchasing, hygiene, and cleaning.

Finally, it is important to start adult service planning early and work with the service/support coordinator or case manager as determined within each state. It may be necessary to apply for funding, be placed on state/county waiting lists, and locate local mental health service options based on each state's provisions and policies.

SUMMARY AND FUTURE DIRECTIONS

Children, adolescents, and adults with ASD/ID and their families require systems of care that provide a range of supports and services throughout the age spectrum and across levels of intensity of challenging behaviors. Most states have studied the increased prevalence of ASD, service needs, and funding streams and have developed response plans. It is the implementation of these plans that requires challenging the institutional, policy, and funding barriers, to create a successful system of care.

REFERENCES

1. Lubetsky MJ, Handen BL, McGonigle JJ, editors. Autism spectrum disorder - Pittsburgh Pocket Psychiatry Series. New York: Oxford University Press, Inc; 2011.
2. Mauch D, Pfefferle S, Booker C, et al. Report on State Services to Individuals with Autism Spectrum Disorder. Centers for Medicare and Medicaid Services, ASD Services Project. 2011. Available at: http://www.cms.gov/apps/files/9-State-Report.pdf. Accessed January 25, 2013.
3. Swiezy NS, Stuwart M, Korzekwa P. Bridging for success in autism: training and collaboration across medical, educational, and community systems. Child Adolesc Psychiatr Clin N Am 2009;17:907–92.
4. Roles for State Title V Programs, Building Systems of Care for Children and Youth with Autism Spectrum Disorder and other Developmental Disabilities, Association of Maternal and Child Health Programs. 2011. Available at: http://www.amchp. org/Calendar/Webinars/ArchivedWebinars/Documents/Full%20Document_Policy %20Framework.pdf. Accessed January 25, 2013.
5. The National Autism Center. National Standards report. 2009. Available at: http:// www.nationalautismcenter.org/pdf/NAC%20NSP%20Report_FIN.pdf. Accessed January 25, 2013.
6. Status Report on Autism Recommendations, The Center for Systems Change. 2012. Available at: http://www.centerforsystemschange.org/view.php?nav_id=46 and http://www.centerforsystemschange.org/up_doc/Status_Report_on_Autism_ Recommendations_5.pdf. Accessed January 25, 2013.
7. Hyman SL, Johnson JK. Autism and pediatric practice: toward a medical home. J Autism Dev Disord 2012;42:1156–64.
8. Autism Screening and Diagnosis for Healthcare Providers, Centers for Disease Control and Prevention. 2012. Available at: http://www.cdc.gov/ncbddd/autism/ hcp-screening.html. Accessed January 25, 2013.
9. Caring for Children With Autism Spectrum Disorders: A Resource Toolkit for Clinicians. American Academy of Pediatrics. 2012, 2007. Available at: http:// www2.aap.org/publiced/autismtoolkit.cfm. Accessed January 25, 2013.
10. Myers SM, Johnson CP. American Academy of Pediatrics, Council on Children With Disabilities. Management of children with autism spectrum disorders. Pediatrics 2007;120(5):1162–82.

11. National Medical Home Autism Initiative. Waisman Center, University of Wisconsin. 2008. Available at: http://www.waisman.wisc.edu/nmhai/. Accessed January 25, 2013.

12. Autism Physician Handbook. Help Autism Now Society (HANS). 2007. Available at: www.helpautismnow.com. Accessed January 25, 2013.

13. Bruder MB, Kerins G, Mazzerella C, et al. Brief report: the medical care of adult with autism spectrum disorders identifying the needs. J Autism Dev Disord 2012; 42:2498–504.

14. Kalb LG, Stuart EA, Freedman B, et al. Psychiatric-related emergency department visits among children with an autism spectrum didorder. Pediatr Emerg Care 2012; 28(12):1269–76.

15. Pennsylvania Autism Task Force Report. 2004. Available at: http://www.dpw.state.pa.us/ucmprd/groups/public/documents/report/s_001624.pdf. Accessed January 25, 2013.

16. Pennsylvania Autism Needs Assessment Report. 2011. Available at: http://www.paautism.org/asert/report.html. Accessed January 25, 2013.

17. Pennsylvania Adult Autism Waiver Program. 2009-2010. Available at: http://www.dpw.state.pa.us/provider/waiverinformation/adultautismwaiver/index.htm. Accessed January 25, 2013.

18. Pennsylvania Adult Community Autism Program (ACAP). 2010. Available at: http://www.dpw.state.pa.us/foradults/autismservices/adultcommunityautismprogramacap/S_000935. Accessed January 25, 2013.

19. Autism in California, 2012 Survey, Autism Society of California. 2012. Available at: https://autismsocietyca.org/uploads/ASC_Survey_April_2012.pdf. Accessed January 25, 2013.

20. HANDS in Autism® Interdisciplinary Training and Resource Center. Christian Sarkine Autism Treatment Center at Riley Hospital at IU Health and the IU School of Medicine. 2008. Available at: www.handsinautism.org. Accessed January 25, 2013.

21. Missouri Rapid Response Project. 2012. Available at: http://dmh.mo.gov/dd/autism/rapidresponse.htm and Thompson Center for Autism. Available at: http://thompsoncenter.missouri.edu/morr/MORR.php. Accessed January 25, 2013.

22. Discussion of the System Designed to Help Children with Severe Autism Spectrum Disorder in Massachusetts. 2012. Available at: http://www.mcpap.com/pdf/Children%20and%20Youth%20with%20Severe%20Autism%20and%20Special%20Education%20Costs.pdf. Accessed January 25, 2013.

23. New Hampshire Council on Autism Spectrum Disorders: Putting the Pieces Together. 2012. Available at: http://www.asdresourcesnh.org/RESOURCESfamily/FAMILYfiles/Council_on_ASD_BROCHURE_9_1_12.pdf and http://www.nhcouncilonasd.org/. Accessed January 25, 2013.

24. Addressing the Needs of Individuals with Autism Spectrum Disorders in Maryland, Recommendations for a Statewide System of Care, Maryland Commission on Autism. 2012. Available at: http://dhmh.maryland.gov/autism/Documents/FINAL_AUTISM_REPORT_10-5-2012.pdf. Accessed January 25, 2013.

25. Autism Guidebook for Washington State, A Resource for Individuals, Families, and Professionals. 2010. Available at: http://here.doh.wa.gov/materials/autism-guidebook/13_AutismGd_E10L.pdf. Accessed January 25, 2013.

26. An Exploration of Fiscal Resources and Systems Needs Related to Autism Spectrum Disorder Services and Supports in Ohio. 2012. Available at: https://ckm.osu.edu/sitetool/sites/caycipublic/documents/OCALI_ForPrint.pdf. Accessed January 25, 2013.

27. National Conference of State Legislatures. 2012. Insurance coverage for autism. Available at: http://www.ncsl.org/issues-research/health/autism-and-insurance-coverage-state-laws.aspx. Accessed January 25, 2013.

28. Pennsylvania Department of Public Welfare Autism Insurance Fact Sheet. Available at: http://www.dpw.state.pa.us/foradults/autismservices/paautismin suranceact62/autisminsuranceactfactsheet/index.htm. Accessed January 25, 2013.

29. Applying Principles of Managed Care to Autism/Services: Challenges, Opportunities and Lessons Learned, New York Health Plan Association. Autism Services Group of Beacon Family of Companies. 2012. Available at: http://www.nyhpa.org/uploads/news_1928913Fligor-Savin%20presentation.pdf. Accessed January 25, 2013.

30. Lord C, McGee JP, editors. The National Academies. Educating children with autism. Washington, DC: National Academy Press; 2001.

31. Kaczmarek LA, Turner K, Alfieri JB. Early childhood interventions. In: Lubetsky MJ, Handen BL, McGonigle JJ, editors. Autism spectrum disorder - Pittsburgh Pocket Psychiatry Series. New York: Oxford University Press, Inc; 2011. p. 147–71.

32. Individuals with Disabilities Education Act (IDEA) Amendments. 2005. Available at: http://www.nasponline.org/advocacy/IDEACRSAnalysis.pdf. Accessed January 25, 2013.

33. Iovannone R, Dunlap G, Huber H, et al. Effective educational practices for students with autism spectrum disorders. Focus Autism Other Dev Disabl 2003;18(3): 150–65.

34. No Child Left Behind Act of 2001. 2002. Available at: http://www2.ed.gov/policy/elsec/leg/esea02/107-110.pdf. Accessed January 25, 2013.

35. Yell ML, Drasgow E, Lowrey KA. No child left behind and students with autism spectrum disorders. Focus Autism Other Dev Disabl 2005;20(3):130–9.

36. Free Appropriate Public Education (FAPE) for Students With Disabilities: Requirements Under Section 504 of The Rehabilitation Act of 1973. 2010. Available at: http://www2.ed.gov/about/offices/list/ocr/docs/edlite-FAPE504.html. Accessed January 25, 2013.

37. McGonigle JJ, Gregory AM, Lubetsky MJ. Transition-age and adult interventions. In: Lubetsky MJ, Handen BL, McGonigle JJ, editors. Autism spectrum disorder - Pittsburgh Pocket Psychiatry Series. New York: Oxford University Press, Inc; 2011. p. 231–51.

Residential Treatment of Serious Behavioral Disturbance in Autism Spectrum Disorder and Intellectual Disability

Carol Anne McNellis, PsyD[a],*, Todd Harris, PhD[b]

KEYWORDS

- Autism • Intellectual disability • Serious behavioral disturbance
- Residential treatment

KEY POINTS

- The behaviors exhibited by children with autism spectrum disorder/intellectual disability and serious behavioral disturbance (SBD) can be extremely dangerous and complicated to treat.
- Philosophic trends toward "least restrictive" treatment choices have had the unintended effect of stigmatizing residential treatment facilities (RTFs) as an option of last resort.
- In many cases, specialized RTF services should be considered as the first choice of treatment to provide the level of treatment intensity necessary to ameliorate SBD.
- Effective contemporary models of residential treatment provide an evidence-based, comprehensive program model that engages families and community resources in treatment.
- RTF providers need to educate funders and legislators on the treatment benefits and cost effectiveness of specialized, intensive models.

INTRODUCTION

In addition to displaying the core symptoms of autism, many children with autism spectrum disorder (ASD)/intellectual disability (ID) may also present with serious behavioral disturbance (SBD). The behavioral presentation of SBD often manifests as overactivity, tantrums, aggression, and self-injurious behaviors.[1,2] Initial treatment

Funding Sources: Nil.
Conflict of Interest: Nil.
[a] Devereux Pennsylvania Children's ID/D Services, 390 East Boot Road, West Chester, PA 19380, USA; [b] Devereux Pennsylvania, 620 Boot Road, Downingtown, PA 19350, USA
* Corresponding author.
E-mail address: cmcnelli@devereux.org

efforts often begin with home-based and community-based treatment services. At present, residential treatment is often offered only as a last resort when home-based and community-based services fail.[3,4] Opponents of residential treatment often cite poor outcomes and isolation from family as primary reasons for its tarnished reputation.[5,6]

This article, however, challenges the idea that residential treatment for this population should be an option of last resort. Residential treatment facilities (RTFs) can offer many advantages, which include a multidisciplinary professional staff, a continuum of care, and a safe therapy and training space for families and discharge providers. These advantages, combined with the best evidence-based treatment, staff training, and staff supervision interventions can make an RTF the first and optimal choice for treatment. Contemporary proponents of residential treatment are answering critics through development of specialized and intensive models of treatment that show significant promise in ameliorating SBD in children with ASD/ID.

CASE: RESIDENTIAL TREATMENT FOR SERIOUS BEHAVIORAL DISTURBANCE

"Sam" was an 11-year-old boy diagnosed with autism and moderate intellectual disability when he was admitted for residential treatment. Sam's parents reported that his history of physical aggression and self-injurious behaviors became increasingly more intense and frequent as he grew older. Sam had been enrolled in special education classes through his local public school, and was receiving home-bound instruction because of the severity of his behavior in the classroom. The family no longer felt safe taking Sam for trips in the community. Before admission for residential treatment, Sam had been hospitalized twice in a children's psychiatric inpatient unit. The family had received outpatient therapy services when Sam was younger and were receiving sporadic in-home therapy services at the time of evaluation for RTF services.

After admission for residential treatment, the treatment team began a multidisciplinary assessment and the process of identifying discharge service providers for linkage with the residential treatment team. Key assessments used in treatment planning for Sam were communication, functional behavior, and psychiatric. Using the assessment information, the team developed a comprehensive positive behavior support plan. Interventions included intensive functional communication training (including targeting functionally equivalent responses); antecedent modifications of the classroom and residence to support communication and instructional opportunities (including the use of visual supports); rich ratios of positive reinforcement to shape targeted responses; and consistent extinction and de-escalation procedures. Psychiatric medications were also adjusted to target the assessed mental health component of existing concerns. At the beginning of treatment, Sam had one-to-one direct staff support for implementation of his behavior support plan for 16 hours a day; the one-to-one approach was faded as treatment progressed. A clinician was also available in the classroom and residence to oversee staff training, and to monitor data collection, implementation integrity, and treatment plan modifications.

Furthermore, Sam's family was actively involved in his residential treatment. The family received training in all interventions outlined in the communication and positive behavior support plans. Training methods included assistance with environmental modifications in the home, shadowing of professional staff, watching video of their son's routines and interventions, and direct coaching (ie, modeling, guidance, and performance feedback). As a part of discharge planning, the residential treatment team also worked with identified community providers of wrap-around services, training them in the treatment protocols in a similar manner as was provided to the family. The residential team then collaborated with the wrap-around provider to begin Sam's transition back to the family home. Discharge was accomplished through a gradual introduction of Sam into his home and into community outings with his family. The residential team continued to provide both in-person support and clinical expertise to the family and wrap-around provider until Sam was fully integrated back home. Gradual reintroduction into the family home occurred at approximately 6 months into Sam's RTF stay, with fading of RTF services and support occurring during the next 6-month treatment period.

EPIDEMIOLOGY

As it is considered one of the most "restrictive" treatment options, residential treatment for children is often initiated only after all community-based treatment options have failed and/or following one or more psychiatric hospitalizations. Children needing residential treatment constitute less than 1% of the general child population.[7] The most common referral concerns that initiate residential treatment are (1) self-injury, (2) physical aggression, (3) other disruptive and destructive acts, and (4) inability to function in daily activities.[8,9] Although these residential referral concerns are consistent across clinical populations with and without ASD, the child with ASD presenting for residential treatment is likely to have a much more complex diagnostic picture. Levy and colleagues[10] found that developmental disabilities co-occur in approximately 83% of children with autism. About 10% of children with autism are also identified as having Down syndrome, Fragile X syndrome, tuberous sclerosis, and other genetic and chromosomal disorders.[11] In addition, severe internalizing symptoms (anxiety, obsessions, compulsions) and externalizing behaviors (aggression, self-injury) are also more likely to occur in children with ASD than in children without ASD.[1,2,12–14] A study completed by Leyfer and colleagues[1] confirmed the presence of at least one DSM-IV (*Diagnostic and Statistical Manual of Mental Disorders* 4th edition, text revision) Axis I psychiatric diagnosis in 72% of children also diagnosed with autism. Finally, a strong predictive relationship has also been demonstrated between SBD and (1) severity of autism symptoms,[15,16] (2) severity of ID,[16,17] and/ or (3) severity of expressive language delay.[16–18]

RTF BEGINNINGS AND LATER TRENDS

The origins of residential treatment for children can be traced to the late 1940s. The establishment of Franklin Roosevelt's New Deal social programs curtailed the need for large public institutions such as orphanages, schools for the intellectually disabled, and homes for delinquent children. These settings were converted to residential centers providing mental health treatment as support for psychiatric interventions increased.[3,4,6] From the 1950s to the 1970s, RTFs flourished.[6] At this time, little distinction was made between psychiatric hospitals and RTFs.

However, during the 1970s accrediting bodies, professional organizations, and funders established a differentiation between psychiatric hospitals and RTFs. These entities defined hospitals as having a medical/psychiatric model, providing a range of different therapies, and delivering services to those with more serious mental health concerns. RTFs, however, were given a decidedly more ambiguous definition whereby an RTF was identified as any other type of 24-hour facility not licensed as a hospital but providing mental health services.[19] A distinction between hospitals and RTFs succeeded only in defining what residential treatment was not, but failed to establish what residential treatment was. Adding to the lack of clarity of purpose for residential treatment was the wide diversity of clinical populations served, theoretical orientations of programs, size of facilities, and services provided. In general, the only commonalities involved were the reliance by RTFs on "milieu therapy" and "life-space interviews" as change agents, but even these intervention elements were inconsistently applied and poorly defined.[20,21] An additional consequence to the interpretation that RTFs were less advanced than their hospital counterparts was significant reductions in reimbursement rates for residential treatment.[6]

More problems for RTFs arose in the 1980s. RTFs began losing favor as a treatment modality because of the ideological trend toward supporting home-based and community-based treatment options, and the inability of RTFs to adapt rapidly to the altered philosophic and financial realities. The Adoption Assistance and Child Welfare Act of 1980 set the legal standards for family preservation efforts that emphasized home placement. The Act had the unintentional effect of creating a focus on a "continuum of care" with the most desirable treatment option being the "least restrictive" choice. As a result, RTFs often became the treatment of last resort because children in RTFs might be isolated from their homes for long periods of time.[3,4] Adding additional weight to arguments for home-based and community-based care was the Child and Adolescent Service System Project (CASSP). CASSP principles defined systems of care for local communities and also supported treatment in "least restrictive environments," which were, preferably, close to the child's home.[3,22] During this period of shifting philosophies, RTFs were challenged to provide more services, in a shorter period of time, and for the same funding rates. Funders began placing an increased emphasis on family work, aftercare planning, and development of adaptive skills to be accomplished in a shorter period of time than was customary for RTFs. Furthermore, with reimbursement dwindling for long-term psychiatric hospitalizations and more services being developed to treat children first in day-care, outpatient, or home-based settings, RTFs in the 1990s also encountered increasing referrals of more seriously disturbed children.[3,6]

ANSWERING CONCERNS ABOUT THE EFFECTIVENESS OF RTF TREATMENT

The reputation of residential treatment was further tarnished after publication of the landmark Report of the Surgeon General on Mental Health in the late 1990s. In this report, RTFs for children were viewed as having "only weak evidence for their effectiveness."[5(p170)] Following publication of this report, concerns mounted that residential treatment was not an evidence-based practice.[23] Supporting this conclusion were criticisms that residential treatment models offered little agreement on key intervention components, often ignored diagnostic groupings, promoted prolonged lengths of stay, created isolation and estrangement from family and community, and produced poor maintenance and generalization outcomes.[7,24,25]

Even with these concerns, RTFs have remained an essential part of the treatment continuum for children. In the United States approximately 50,000 children a year are admitted to residential treatment.[26] The case of "Sam" (see earlier case discussion) demonstrates how residential treatment can be an effective and efficient service delivery model for children with ASD/ID and SBD. As comprehensive treatment centers with multidisciplinary staff, RTFs can offer many advantages. In addition, newer models for residential treatment are emerging that are designed to address the concerns raised by the critics of residential treatment through adherence to best-practice guidelines for special clinical populations and the development of essential, evidence-based program components.

Advantages of an RTF for Children with ASD/ID and SBD

The comprehensive and multidisciplinary organizational structure of RTFs offers many advantages.

First, RTFs bring together a multitude of skilled, multidisciplinary professionals in one location. Given the complex diagnostic picture of children with ASD/ID and SBD, having specialists in psychiatry, neurology, psychology, behavior analysis, special education, and speech and occupational therapy readily available, and able to work together as a team, is highly beneficial for efficacious treatment.

Second, RTFs are often a part of a continuum of treatment services. Children can step up or down in level of care as needed, with planning and transfer accomplished smoothly by the same provider of services. For example, a campus-based RTF may plan for a step down to a facility-owned community-based RTF or group home as an interim step before discharge home.

Third, RTFs can offer a safe space for in vivo parent training. Parents of children with ASD/ID and SBD can be despairing and exhausted by the time their child is admitted for residential treatment. Parent training within the RTF setting, however, provides the space where parents can observe staff working successfully with their child. Parents can then practice the same interventions with professionals on hand to coach, provide feedback, and reinforce successful implementation in both the RTF environment and the family home.

Fourth, RTFs can provide the space and staff to train aftercare providers to replicate interventions when the child returns home. While some RTF providers are also developing their own community-based service providers for aftercare, the ability of an RTF to train any aftercare provider in the treatment interventions is a decided plus, especially in rural areas where individuals skilled in working with children with ASD/ID may be limited.

Evidence-Based Interventions and Practices

Residential treatment has suffered since its inception from vague definitions of program model components and agents of change. Proponents of residential treatment, however, have frequently criticized studies reporting on the ineffectiveness of residential treatment because of the lack of consensus as to what the studies were actually measuring. Almost all of the studies compared the effectiveness of RTFs based only on the setting where treatment was delivered, without comparing the different treatment components within the setting. These studies demonstrate that there is little research that can definitively tell us what is effective or ineffective about residential treatment.[6,27,28] Newer RTF models, however, focus on delivery of evidence-based interventions and practices within the RTF setting. Because there is a strong evidence base already established for the interventions, these components of treatment should be portable from setting to setting if delivered with integrity.[3]

In recent years, there has been increasing documentation of effective intervention practices for individuals with autism that are supported by empirical research. For example, the National Standards Report[29] reviewed and analyzed 775 peer-reviewed research articles. Each intervention was then grouped into 1 of 4 different categories: Established (effective interventions that were supported by reviewed research); Emerging (interventions that show promise by one or more studies, but do not meet the criteria for Established); Unestablished (interventions with little or no support from empirical evidence); and Ineffective/Harmful (research has demonstrated that these interventions are not effective and/or can lead to harm). In 2007, the Office of Special Education Programs in the US Department of Education funded a similar endeavor by the National Professional Development Center on Autism Spectrum Disorders. The outcome of this project was the identification of 24 practices that met predetermined criteria for evidence-based practices for children and youth with ASDs.[30] In 2009, Maine's Department of Health and Human Services, in conjunction with the State Department of Education, also produced a report outlining levels of empirical support for various interventions for children with an ASD.[31] Although there were some minor differences in the findings produced in these documents, most of their conclusions regarding interventions were largely consistent. All 3 reports suggest that interventions based on the principles of applied behavior analysis (ABA) are the most effective in producing favorable outcomes.

While these reports have provided guidance to clinicians, educators, and families when determining the best course of intervention, there have been no such reports outlining best practice specifically for RTFs based on meta-analysis reviews.[3] Nevertheless, it is thought that these interventions and best practices are not typically setting specific, and would consequently apply to RTFs. Therefore, the following briefly reviews proposed best-practice strategies and essential program components for RTFs serving children and adolescents with an ASD or ID (extrapolated from the findings documented in the previously mentioned reports as well as other findings).

Best-Practice Strategies

The use of ABA instructional methods

As discussed previously, ABA instructional strategies are widely supported as effective for children and adolescents with an ASD or ID.[29] Indeed, research has shown that ABA is effective for teaching communication skills,[32,33] social skills,[34,35] and skills related to independent living.[36,37]

On completion of a comprehensive skills assessment, an instructional plan is typically developed for each targeted skill. Although there is some variation among different organizations, most ABA-based instructional summaries contain the following.[38,39]

- *Goal statements and behavioral objectives* that operationally define the targeted skill, define the conditions under which it should be emitted, and define (observable and measurable) criteria for mastery.
- *A system for providing and fading prompts* that includes the types of prompts to be used and the process for introduction and fading (eg, prompt hierarchy, prompt fading, delayed prompts, or graduated guidance).
- *A system for providing differential reinforcement* that includes a reward menu based on the outcomes of a structured preference assessment, visual mediation of reinforcement contingencies, and a plan to gradually thin reinforcement and build natural reinforcement contingencies.
- *A plan on how to best arrange the lessons* that includes such options as discrete trial training, incidental teaching, chaining, and shaping. As part of each lesson, there should also be a planned way to respond to (and correct) errors.
- *A plan on how to promote skill generalization and maintenance* that includes procedures that enhance generalization across people (professional staff, families, community contacts), settings (home, school, community), and situations/materials.
- *Procedures for data collection and analysis* that outline operational definitions, how data will be collected, who will collect data and how frequently, and who analyzes the data and reports on progress. There must also be a mechanism that ensures that decisions related to modifying each instructional summary are data driven.

Environmental milieu expectations

Newer RTF models are finding success narrowing their focus by concentrating treatment efforts on very specific target populations such as children and adolescents with ASD/ID and SBD. By addressing the needs of a specific clinical population, RTFs can develop an uninterrupted "milieu" where every staff interaction, activity, and even the living space supports the specific treatment needs of the target population.[3] Furthermore, the treatment outcomes of ABA instructional methods can be enhanced when implemented in a structured and supportive context such as an RTF. The following are some program components and characteristics that are thought to be essential for optimal treatment response.

Predictable and structured routines with high engagement levels Research has shown that predictability and high levels of child engagement lead to increased skill acquisition and reduced behavioral issues.[40] These effects can be further enhanced when individuals have frequent choices and when preferences are incorporated into routines.[41]

Functional communication and social skills training Paramount to the long-term success for individuals with ASD/ID is the acquisition of essential communication and social skills. Teaching targets in these areas must be based on each individual's specific deficits, with consideration of their needs in present and future settings. Instruction must be intensive and structured, and must to be embedded into routines across all settings to optimize skill generalization and maintenance.[42,43]

Use of visual supports Learning can also be enhanced through the use of visual support strategies. Visual supports are most commonly used for schedules, choice making, reinforcement systems, and learning sequenced tasks. These strategies are also frequently used when teaching communication and social skills.[33,36,37,44,45]

Errorless learning Frequent errors during learning can slow acquisition and increase rates of problematic behavior.[46] Therefore, instruction should be designed to limit the number of errors whenever possible (typically accomplished through prompt fading and/or shaping procedures).

Community-based instruction Despite attempts by families to teach community skills, many children with an ASD or ID continue to have great difficulty in community settings (both behaviorally and through not having the skills needed to be independent in these settings). An absence of these critical skills can often lead to child and/or family isolation, and will greatly affect an individual's quality of life as he or she enters adulthood. However, specialized and frequent training in community skills will lead to acquisition (and/or generalization) of these skills[47] and a reduction in behaviors that interfere with successful community inclusion.

Essential Program Components

In addition to implementing best practices related to instruction and environmental milieu expectations, other related program components are necessary to achieve the desired goal of generalized and durable treatment gains in residential treatment facilities. The following describe some of these components.

Family inclusion, engagement, and training

A frequently voiced concern about residential treatment is the fear that children may be unnecessarily isolated from their families. Newer models of RTF for children begin with active family engagement and discharge planning at admission. From the onset, it is critical that families are considered partners in treatment and are actively involved in the assessment and planning processes, as well being trained to implement intervention strategies.[48] One approach strongly supported by empirical research, Behavioral Parent Training, teaches family members to use ABA teaching strategies with their child in home and community settings.[49,50] This approach has led to family members being able to effectively manage their child's behaviors while also teaching new skills. However, similar to outcomes found in staff training, some form of ongoing, in-home performance feedback and other forms of support (ie, modeling, coaching) will likely be necessary for durable change in family skills.[51]

Individualized positive behavior support processes

To successfully treat challenging and dangerous responses, it is imperative that there is an understanding of why a behavior is occurring (ie, the function or functions of a behavior). In other words, professionals and family members need to identify the antecedents that are associated with higher response rates, as well as the consequences that are maintaining these rates. This understanding, accomplished through completion of a Functional Behavior Assessment (FBA) or Functional Analysis, should then serve as the foundation of a comprehensive Positive Behavior Support (PBS) plan.

The emphasis of the PBS plan will then be to prevent (or reduce) the occurrence of unwanted responses by modifying the instructional and social environments; teaching pro-social responses that serve the same function as the unwanted responses; and the use of differential reinforcement contingencies to increase desired responding. Consequences following the unwanted responses should focus on avoiding or minimizing the amount of reinforcement obtained while keeping the individual and others safe. Objective data are used to determine if the plan is working and to guide decisions regarding necessary modifications. Close coordination and continuous communication among professional staff (ie, physicians, psychiatrists, behavior analysts/psychologists, and educators) and the family is important in maximizing the positive impact of the PBS plan.

Staff training and supervision

To deliver the evidence-based interventions necessary to ensure treatment success, residential and community-based direct support staff must have adequate training in ASDs, ABA instructional strategies, functional communication interventions, and implementation of PBS plans. Training workshops are the first necessary step in the professional development process, but research has illustrated that workshops alone rarely lead to improved and durable changes in staff performance. Therefore, it is critical that other effective strategies be implemented to optimize staff performance. These "behavioral supervision" strategies may include modeling and coaching, performance feedback, and goal setting.[52–54]

Intensive treatment services

Some of the most successful contemporary models of RTF offer treatment services that are delivered more intensively than older models. By delivering therapy services more frequently to both the individual and family, lengths of stay can be significantly shortened. RTF direct care staff members are expected to be active participants in treatment, providing direct observation feedback, carrying out treatment protocols with fidelity, and documenting interventions and child response. This level of focused treatment often requires one-to-one direct care staffing ratios during the early stages of treatment. Intensive RTFs also require an increase in clinical oversight to enable clinicians to manage smaller caseloads. However, with the increased staffing support also comes more accountability for ensuring intensive, active treatment that is congruent with an evidence-based program model.[6,27,55]

Comprehensive discharge planning

Comprehensive discharge planning that begins at admission provides the framework to ensure that all necessary support and treatment services are identified and are in place at the time of discharge. The RTF provider can provide case-management services or work with a local mental health, ID, or ASD case manager to identify the type and intensity of treatment services needed to support the child's return home. Critical to this process is provision of overlap of services between the RTF provider and the community provider. The overlap supports continuity of care by allowing the community team to become familiar with the child, family, and RTF treatment plan while the child is still receiving RTF treatment.[56] Further, comprehensive discharge planning also involves identifying important community resources to support the overall transition of the child back to the home setting. Important resources to identify include school and after-school programs, extended family support, recreational activities, and respite services.[48]

SUMMARY AND FUTURE DIRECTIONS

For children with ASD/ID who also exhibit SBD, specialized (ie, autism/ID-specific assessments and interventions) and intensive residential treatment may be the most effective and efficient treatment option. The case example earlier in this article demonstrates how an evidenced-based, autism-specific treatment model can be applied successfully in an RTF by using the integrated professional resources of the setting, state-of-the-science assessments and interventions, and an intensive method of service delivery. The case example also demonstrates 2 other important points for consideration in the discussion about the treatment needs of this special clinical population.

First, because there has been considerable research supporting home-based and community-based treatment models, residential treatment is often relegated to "the treatment of last resort." Children are not placed in RTFs until all lesser restrictive options have been tried and failed, setting up an unfortunate and potentially dangerous situation whereby children must drop out of all other service delivery systems before they can be referred to an appropriate level of care. Frequently, years of valuable treatment time are wasted, and financial resources are directed toward levels of care that are insufficient for treating severe and complex behavioral issues. Residential treatment deserves to be considered a viable and equal partner in the continuum of community service systems.[3] Furthermore, by recognizing the value of residential treatment in the continuum of care, individuals can move more seamlessly into and out of the level of care needed, as often as needed, without the stigma of somehow having "failed" by needing the level of care provided by RTFs.[6]

Second, Sam was diagnosed in early childhood with autism, ID, and clear and significant communication deficits. As discussed previously, there is a strong predictive relationship between SBD and the combination of autism, ID, and expressive language delay. If a child is diagnosed early in life with even one of the predictive triad of symptoms, studies have demonstrated that early intensive intervention services that combine speech and language therapy, proactive, PBS interventions, and parent training can be an effective preventive measure in the development of severe problem behaviors.[57,58] Although considerable funding and attention has been expended in development of home-based and community-based interventions to address well-established behavioral concerns, more consideration needs to be focused on preventive interventions for this diagnostic group. Early, intensive intervention has shown great potential for averting the development of SBD in all but the most difficult cases. If diagnosis can occur early, and intensive services are begun at the time of diagnosis, the majority of these children may never need residential treatment services.

As newer models of residential treatment continue to evolve, those serving children with ASD/ID and SBD will need to concentrate their efforts in improving services with a focus on these areas.

Funding

Many RTF providers face a shortfall of funding because of outdated funder perceptions, which fail to recognize that the increased acuity level of referrals combined with the complexity of the diagnostic concerns creates the need for more intensive services and, therefore, more costly services. Furthermore, because of misconceptions regarding the effectiveness of residential treatment, many state and local agencies have cut funding for residential treatment.[27] Also adding to the financial strain on RTFs was the movement toward more home-based and community-based services, which served not only to develop the philosophy of "least restrictive" care but also was seen as a "less expensive" treatment choice in comparison with residential treatment. The idea of cost containment opened the door to managed care funding for all mental health service delivery systems. Early efforts at cost containment by managed care funders virtually wiped out residential capacities in many areas, as a result of well-intentioned but misguided efforts to limit lengths of stay unnecessarily and failure to maintain the necessary range of RTF services for children and families. However, newer funding models for residential treatment are finding success by partnering with funders to develop more intensive service models within a flexible system of care. Many of these models can also allow for overlap of services between levels of care.[3,56] To establish the partnership, current residential providers must advocate with funders and legislators for adequate financial resources to meet the intensive treatment needs of children with ASD/ID and SBD. When making the case for higher rates with funders, residential providers must arm themselves with the research that demonstrates the effectiveness of intensive intervention, and data supporting the cost-effectiveness of intervening with the right level of care early in the treatment process.

Intensive Case-Management Services

As previously discussed, children with ASD/ID and SBD have complex service and treatment needs. Along with the need for early identification and intervention is the need for intensive case-management services. Because of the specialized nature of the support needed, families often require assistance in finding these services. As a child's special needs are identified, ideally an intensive case manager would identify and link the family to a myriad of services to address the educational, mental health/behavioral, speech, recreational, respite, employment, and housing needs that surround a diagnosis of ASD/ID.

Family Intervention

Often, the biggest barriers to family intervention when a child is placed in an RTF are time and distance. Because specialized RTFs do not exist in every local community, the closest specialized RTF for a family may be several hours away from the home. Specialized RTF providers must be flexible and creative to overcome these barriers. Clinical and other treatment staff will need to be available to families on evenings and weekends when the parents have time to participate in treatment. Creative use of technology can also assist in overcoming time and distance barriers. Videotaping staff implementing a treatment protocol or assisting a child through a daily routine can be a valuable training tool for families. Use of Skype and other technology to facilitate parent coaching sessions and deliver performance feedback is increasingly being used to break down barriers of time and distance. Technology can be used not only to train families but also to train local providers of community services who will be responsible for aftercare services.[49]

Community Involvement

RTF providers must also offer treatment planning with a focus on substantial community inclusion and training efforts. Treatment settings must extend outside the RTF walls to those community venues where the child should be successful so as to reintegrate into his or her family's daily life. Instruction should be delivered in settings that the family frequently patronizes (ie, grocery stores, parks, malls, restaurants, and so forth) to generalize skills learned beyond the RTF setting. Parents must be involved in the community training sessions to gain both skills and confidence working with their child in familiar community environments. Without significant attention to community inclusion and training efforts, RTFs will continue to suffer criticism about maintenance and generalization failures.

In conclusion, as professionals continue to pursue the most effective methods of improving the lives of individuals with ASD/ID who have an SBD, RTFs can be a critical treatment tool in the portfolio of services needed to address the complex challenges of this population. However, a successful RTF must be grounded in an intensive treatment model that focuses on the use of ABA instructional strategies to teach communication, social, independent living, and community skills. FBA data must guide the development of PBS plans, and staff must be properly trained and supervised in implementing these plans with a high degree of fidelity.

For intervention gains to generalize to home and community settings, as well as to be maintained over time, families must be involved from the very beginning of treatment and throughout the process. Furthermore, families need to be trained to implement successful interventions and receive support in the form of intervention modeling, coaching, and performance feedback. These activities, along with intensive case-management services and comprehensive discharge planning, will further enhance the possibilities of desirable long-term outcomes.

Finally, as the technology for effective treatment of this population evolves, it will be necessary to reconsider how funding is arranged. Although this intensive model may be more expensive initially, recent studies with other populations suggest that lengths of stay will be shorter and readmission rates to RTFs decreased.[56] Therefore, this model can be more cost-effective and produce more optimal and durable outcomes than the traditional RTF models.

REFERENCES

1. Leyfer OT, Folstein SE, Bacalman S, et al. Comorbid psychiatric disorders in children with autism: interview development and rates of disorders. J Autism Dev Disord 2006;36:849–61.
2. Lecavalier L. Behavioral and emotional problems in young people with pervasive developmental disorders: relative prevalence, effects of subject characteristics, and empirical classification. J Autism Dev Disord 2006;36:1101–14.
3. Lieberman RE. Future directions in residential treatment. Child Adolesc Psychiatr Clin N Am 2004;13:279–94.
4. Small R. Charting a new course. Contributions to residential treatment. Washington, DC: American Association of Children's Residential Centers; 2003. p. 72–6.
5. Department of Health and Human Services. Mental health: a report of the surgeon general. Profiles in science: National Library of Medicine. Available at: http://profiles.nlm.nih.gov/ps/retrieve/ResourceMetadata/NNBBHS. Published 1999. Updated April 9, 2002. Accessed December 12, 2012.
6. Leichtman M. Residential treatment of children and adolescents: past, present, and future. Am J Orthopsychiatry 2006;6(3):285–94.

7. Whittaker JK. The re-invention of residential treatment: an agenda for research and practice. Child Adolesc Psychiatr Clin N Am 2004;13(2):267–78.

8. Abt Associates Inc. Characteristics of residential treatment for children and youth with serious emotional disturbance. National Association of Psychiatric Health Systems; 2008. Available at: www.naphs.org/documents/AbtFINALReport. Accessed November 19, 2012.

9. McCurdy BL, McIntyre EK. "And what about residential...?" Re-conceptualizing residential treatment as a stop-gap service for youth with emotional and behavioral disorders. Behav Interv 2004;19(3):137–58.

10. Levy SE, Giarelli E, Lee L, et al. Autism spectrum disorder and co-occurring developmental, psychiatric, and medical conditions among children in multiple populations of the United States. J Dev Behav Pediatr 2010;31(4):267–75.

11. Centers for Disease Control and Prevention. Autism spectrum disorders (ASD's): data and statistics. Centers for Disease Control and Prevention; 2012. Available at: http://www.cdc.gov/ncbddd/autism/data.html. Accessed December 6, 2012.

12. Hartley SL, Sikora DM, McCoy R. Prevalence and risk factors of maladaptive behaviour in young children with autistic disorder. J Intellect Disabil Res 2008; 52(10):819–29.

13. Gadow KD, DeVincent CJ, Pomeroy J, et al. Psychiatric symptoms in preschool children with PDD and clinic and comparison samples. J Autism Dev Disord 2004;34(4):379–93.

14. Gadow KD. Comparison of DSM-IV symptoms in elementary school-age children with PDD versus clinic and community samples. Autism 2005;9(4): 392–415.

15. Jang J, Dixon DR, Tarbox J, et al. Symptom severity and challenging behavior in children with ASD. Res Autism Spectr Disord 2011;5(3):1028–32.

16. Dominick KC, Davis NO, Lainhart J, et al. Atypical behaviors in children with autism and children with a history of language impairment. Res Dev Disabil 2007;28(2):145–62.

17. De Bildt A, Sytema S, Kraijer D, et al. Adaptive functioning and behavior problems in relation to level of education in children and adolescents with intellectual disability. J Intellect Disabil Res 2005;49:672–81.

18. Durand V. Functional communication training using assistive devices: effects on challenging behavior and affect. Augment Altern Commun 1993;9(3):168–76.

19. Tuma JM. Mental health services for children: the state of the art. Am Psychol 1989;44(2):188–99.

20. Whittaker JK. Developing a unified theory of residential treatment. Ment Hyg 1970;54:166–9.

21. Trieschman AE, Whittaker JK, Brendtro LK. The other 23 hours: child-care work with emotionally disturbed children in a therapeutic milieu. New York: Aldine De Gruyter; 1969.

22. Stroul BA, Friedman RM. A system of care for seriously emotionally disturbed children and youth. Washington, DC: Georgetown University Child Development Center, CASSP Technical Assistance Center; 1986.

23. Hoagwood K, Burns B, Kiser L, et al. Evidenced based practice in child and adolescent mental health services. Psychiatr Serv 2001;52(9):1179–89.

24. Lebuffe PA, Robison S, Chamberlin-Elliott DA. Residential treatment centers for children and adolescents with conduct disorders. In: Murrihy RC, Kidman AD, Ollendick TH, editors. Clinical handbook of assessing and treating conduct problems in youth. New York: Springer; 2010. p. 333–64.

25. Burns BJ, Hoagwood K, Mrazek P. Effective treatment for mental disorders in children and adolescents. Clin Child Fam Psychol Rev 1999;2:199–254.
26. Vaughn CF. Residential treatment centers: not a solution for children with mental health needs. Clearinghouse Review Journal of Poverty Law and Policy 2005; 39(3–4):274.
27. Butler LS, McPherson PM. Is residential treatment misunderstood? J Child Fam Stud 2007;16(4):465–72.
28. Hair HJ. Outcomes for children and adolescents after residential treatment: a review of research from 1993 to 2003. J Child Fam Stud 2005;14(4):551–75.
29. National Autism Center. National standards report. Available at: http://www.nationalautismcenter.org/nsp/reports.php. Published 2009. Accessed December 12, 2012.
30. The National Professional Development Center on Autism Spectrum Disorders. Evidence based practices briefs. Available at: http://autismpdc.fpg.unc.edu/content/evidence-based-practices. Published 2010. Accessed December 12, 2012.
31. Maine Department of Health and Human Services and the Maine Department of Education. Interventions for autism spectrum disorders: state of the evidence. Available at: muskie.usm.maine.edu/Publications/cutler/autism-spectrum-disorders-report2009.pdf. Published October 2009. Accessed December 2, 2012.
32. Charlop MH, Carpenter MH. Modified incidental teaching sessions: procedure for parents to increase spontaneous speech in their children with autism. J Posit Behav Interv 2000;2(2):98–112.
33. Charlop-Christy MH, Kelso SE. Teaching children with autism conversational speech using a cue card/written script program. Educ Treat Children 2003; 26(2):108–27.
34. Krantz PJ, McClannahan LE. Social interaction skills for children with autism: a script-fading procedure for beginning readers. J Appl Behav Anal 1998;31(2): 191–202.
35. Pierce KL, Schreibman L. Multiple peers use of pivotal response training to increase social behaviors of classmates with autism: results from trained and untrained peers. J Appl Behav Anal 1997;30(1):157–60.
36. MacDuff GS, Krantz PJ, McClannahan LE. Teaching children with autism to use photographic activity schedules: maintenance and generalization of complex response chains. J Appl Behav Anal 1993;26(1):89–97.
37. Pierce KL, Schreibman L. Teaching daily living skills to children with autism in unsupervised settings through pictorial self-management. J Appl Behav Anal 1994;27:471–81.
38. Cooper JO, Heron TE, Heward WL. Applied behavior analysis. 2nd edition. Upper Saddle River (NJ): Pearson; 2007.
39. Sulzer-Azaroff B, Mayer GR. Behavior analysis for lasting change. Orlando (FL): Holt Rinehart & Winston; 1991.
40. O'Reilly M, Sigafoos J, Lancioni G, et al. An examination of the effects of a classroom activity schedule on levels of self-Injury and engagement for a child with severe autism. J Autism Dev Disord 2005;35:305–11.
41. Dyer K, Dunlap G, Winterling V. Effects of choice making on the serious problem behaviors of students with severe handicaps. J Appl Behav Anal 1990;23(4): 515–24.
42. Bellini S, Peters JK, Brenner L, et al. A meta-analysis of school-based social skills interventions for children with autism spectrum disorders. Remedial Spec Educ 2007;28(3):153–62.

43. Gresham FM, Sugai G, Horner RH. Interpreting outcomes of social skills training for students with high-incidence disabilities. Teaching Exceptional Children 2001;67:331–44.

44. Johnston S, Nelson C, Evans J, et al. The use of visual supports in teaching young children with autism spectrum disorder to initiate interactions. Augment Altern Commun 2003;19:86–104.

45. Wantanabe M, Sturmey P. The effect of choice-making opportunities during activity schedules on task engagement of adults with autism. J Autism Dev Disord 2003;33(5):535–8.

46. Gaylord-Ross R. Task difficulty and aberrant behavior in severely handicapped students. J Appl Behav Anal 1981;14:449–63.

47. Alcantara PR. Effects of videotape instructional package on purchasing skills of children with autism. Except Children 1994;61(1):40–55.

48. Magellan Lehigh Valley Care Management Center. One-year outcomes report: short-term residential treatment facility (RTF) pilot program. Magellan Health Services; 2010. Available at: http://www.magellanofpa.com/media/157075/lehigh%20short%20term%20rtf_final.pdf. Accessed December 12, 2012.

49. Symon JB. Providing parent education for autism: issues in providing services at a distance. J Posit Behav Interv 2001;3:160–74.

50. Symon JB. Expanding interventions for children with autism: parents as trainers. J Posit Behav Interv 2005;7:159–73.

51. Harris TA, Peterson SL, Filliben T, et al. Evaluating a more cost-efficient alternative to providing in-home feedback to parents: the use of spousal feedback. J Appl Behav Anal 1998;31(1):131–4.

52. Parsons MB, Reid DH. Training residential supervisors to provide feedback for maintaining staff teaching skills with people who have severe disabilities. J Appl Behav Anal 1995;28:317–22.

53. Reid DF, Parson MB, Greene CW. The supervisor training curriculum for developmental disability organizations—evidence-based ways to promote work quality and enjoyment among support staff. Washington, DC: American Association on Intellectual and Developmental Disabilities; 2011.

54. Dyer K, Schwartz IS, Luce SC. A supervision program for increasing functional activities for severely handicapped students in a residential setting. J Appl Behav Anal 1984;17:249–59.

55. Leichtman M, Leichtman ML, Barber CC, et al. Effectiveness of intensive short-term residential treatment with severely disturbed adolescents. Am J Orthopsychiatry 2001;71(2):227–35.

56. Magellan Health Services Children's Services Task Force. Perspectives on residential and community-based treatment of youth and families. Magellan Health Services; 2008. Avaliable at: http://www.magellanhealth.com/media/2718/CommunityResidentailTreatmentWhitePaper.pdf. Accessed December 1, 2012.

57. Jacobson JW, Mulick JA. System and cost research issues in treatment for people with autistic disorders. J Autism Dev Disord 2000;30(6):585–93.

58. Ruble LA, Heflinger CA, Renfrew JW, et al. Access and service use by children with autism spectrum disorders in Medicaid managed care. J Autism Dev Disord 2005;35(1):3–13.

Psychiatric Hospital Treatment of Children with Autism and Serious Behavioral Disturbance

Matthew Siegel, MD[a],*, Robin L. Gabriels, PsyD[b]

KEYWORDS

- Inpatient • Autism • Intellectual disability • Hospitalization • Psychiatric

KEY POINTS

- Eleven percent of children with autism spectrum disorder (ASD) are admitted to a psychiatric hospital unit before adulthood.
- Children with ASD are admitted primarily because of externalizing behaviors: aggression, self-injury, and tantrums.
- Externalizing behaviors frequently represent a manifestation of impaired emotion regulation or acute exacerbation of a comorbid psychiatric disorder.
- Successful management requires a broad multidisciplinary diagnostic approach that manages acute symptoms and ameliorates key perpetuating factors, such as sleep deprivation, communication inefficiency, or environmental reinforcement of maladaptive behaviors.
- There is preliminary evidence for the effectiveness of specialized hospital psychiatry units designed for the ASD and intellectual disability population, and there is a lack of studies of general psychiatric hospital treatment of this population.

INTRODUCTION

Children with an autism spectrum disorder (ASD) are admitted to psychiatric hospitals at high rates, but some institutions refuse or are unable to serve them. This paradox springs from the application of a brief inpatient intervention model initially developed for the neurotypical population to children with ASD. The ASD population has unique abilities and needs and typically presents with externalizing behaviors that require intensive assessment and intervention methods to tease out the underlying issues fueling the crisis presentation.

The authors report no financial disclosures or conflicts of interest.
[a] Developmental Disorders Program, Maine Medical Center Research Institute, Tufts University School of Medicine, Spring Harbor Hospital, 123 Andover Road, Westbrook, ME 04096, USA;
[b] Neuropsychiatric Special Care Program, Children's Hospital Colorado, University of Colorado Denver Anschutz Medical Campus, 13123 East 16th Avenue, Aurora, CO 80045, USA
* Corresponding author.
E-mail address: siegem@springharbor.org

Admission to psychiatric hospitals of children with ASD or intellectual disability (ID) creates a separation from family, educational services, and therapeutic programming, as well as substantial financial costs. Despite the impacts of frequent admissions on public health and caregivers, there is little information in the scientific literature regarding psychiatric hospital treatment of this population. Hospitalization is usually based on acutely unsafe behaviors, which can be generated by impaired emotion regulation, behavioral excesses, and/or comorbid psychiatric illness. Children with ASD and/or ID have higher rates of comorbid psychiatric illness than the general pediatric population.[1,2] Children with ASD and ID also show delays in social communication skills and the development of emotion regulation. These characteristics can lead to bullying or exclusion from peer groups, social isolation, suspension from school and communication frustration, all of which can increase the risk of developing comorbid psychiatric illness and/or acute behavioral disturbance.

To facilitate best practices for this population, this article (1) presents the evidence for inpatient treatment of ASD in both general and specialized child psychiatry units, (2) outlines approaches to inpatient treatment of this population, and (3) describes 2 specialized hospital programs designed for the ASD and ID populations.

EPIDEMIOLOGY, COSTS, AND ACCESS

Eleven percent of children with ASD are reported by their parents to have been psychiatrically hospitalized in the United States by 21 years of age.[3] The 1-year prevalence of psychiatric hospitalization of children with ASD is 1.3% to 7.0%.[3,4] By comparison, only 0.23% of privately insured children in the United States were psychiatrically hospitalized in the year 2000.[5]

Two large studies have examined psychiatric hospital admission rates for children with ASD. Among 760 children with ASD aged 5 to 21 years, the strongest predictors of psychiatric hospitalization were the following:[3]

- Aggressive behavior (odds ratio [OR] = 4.83)
- Coming from a single-parent home (OR = 2.54)
- Depression (OR = 2.48)
- Obsessive compulsive disorder (OCD) (OR = 2.35)
- Self-injurious behavior (OR = 2.14)

Risk for hospitalization increased over time and with patient age. Additionally, caregivers of psychiatrically hospitalized youth had a lower socioeconomic status and educational attainment than those whose children had not experienced hospitalization. Another large study of 33,000 children aged 2 to 18 years revealed a ratio of 6.6 ASD psychiatric admissions to every one non-ASD psychiatric admission. Even more striking, the children with ASD incurred 11.9 times more psychiatric hospital days, indicating that children with ASD also have longer hospital stays on average. A recent study of almost 4 million emergency department visits in the United States found that 13% of children with ASD who presented to the emergency department were there for mental health problems; comparatively, only 2% of non-ASD children came for such problems.[6]

A few protective factors associated with a lower risk of psychiatric hospitalization in the ASD population have been identified; these factors include living in an area with a high number of pediatric specialists, being female, younger age, and using respite care.[7] In particular, every $1000 increase in spending on respite care during the preceding 60 days resulted in an 8% decrease in the odds of hospitalization. However, as the investigators point out, aggressive or self-injurious behaviors, the primary reasons for psychiatric hospitalization, may disqualify children from receiving respite care. Because respite care is not typically thought of as a treatment for children with ASD, it is not yet known if providing respite care lowers total psychiatric hospitalization over time or simply delays it.

The cost of psychiatric hospitalization is a large component of the total health care costs for individuals with ASD. In a comparison study, children with ASD incurred 12.4 times the cost for psychiatric hospitalization than children without ASD.[4] Additionally, 10% of the children with ASD accounted for 53% of the total annual cost of medical care, and almost all of the children with ASD who had been psychiatrically hospitalized were in the highest decile for total health care costs.

If we extrapolate a conservative 1.3% 1-year prevalence of psychiatric hospitalization to the estimated 760,000 children with ASD in the United States (1% of 76 million children), up to 10,000 children with ASD are psychiatrically hospitalized each year. As children with ASD have been identified in increasing numbers by the Centers for Disease Control and Prevention[8] and psychiatric hospitalization costs for ASD increase with age,[9,10] psychiatric hospitalization costs will likely swell over the coming decade.

Although the psychiatric hospitalization of children with ASD is prevalent, there are multiple barriers to care that can perpetuate a state of crisis for this population. Stigma associated with developmental disorders is reflected in the rules of some health insurers, which require that an individual with ASD must also have a comorbid psychiatric illness in order to access psychiatric hospital care. The logic of such rule making is difficult to discern, considering that no other group with a *Diagnostic and Statistical Manual of Mental Disorders* (Fourth Edition, Text Revision)[11] axis I psychiatric disorder is required to have an additional axis I disorder to access treatment.

Conversely, insurers and some practitioners can fall victim to diagnostic overshadowing,[12] ascribing all facets of a child's presentation (aggression, self-injury, and change in sleep patterns) to the background ASD or ID diagnosis rather than to a possible comorbid disorder. This error of attribution is then conflated with a presumption that the symptoms are chronic and untreatable, leading to a circular justification for denial of care. It is simply not normal or typical, however, for children with ASD to repeatedly strike themselves or others and to suggest otherwise represents a lack of knowledge and/or an ethical failure in the service of cost containment.

Stigma can also affect the willingness of institutions and clinicians to provide psychiatric hospital care to individuals with ASD or ID; therefore, access to inpatient care varies widely across institutions. Notably, a study of *boarding* in a pediatric emergency department, a term for staying in the emergency department while awaiting a psychiatric hospital bed, found that having a diagnosis of ASD was the number one predictor of boarding, followed by having an ID diagnosis.[13] In addition, most child psychiatry trainees see less than 5 outpatients and 10 inpatients with ASD or ID per year during their 2 years of training.[14] This very limited clinical exposure has particularly concerning implications for inpatient treatment, given that child psychiatric hospital units are almost universally led by child psychiatrists.

RECENT DEVELOPMENTS IN PSYCHIATRIC HOSPITAL CARE FOR CHILDREN WITH ASD

Psychiatric hospital treatment of individuals with ASD and/or ID has developed from the earlier twentieth century era of long-term institutionalization, through the movement for deinstitutionalization and normalization of the 1970s and 1980s, to the current era of short-stay acute admissions.

Most hospitalized children with ASD in the United States are treated in general child psychiatry units. However, over the last decade, the number of *specialized* hospital psychiatry units (those that exclusively serve children with ASD or ID) has doubled in the United States.[15] A recent survey identified 9 of these units in the United States. These units universally used a combined pharmacologic and behavioral therapy approach, used large multidisciplinary treatment teams (average of 4.6 disciplines), and had an average length of stay of 42.3 days. The most common chief admission complaint was aggression, followed by self-injurious behavior, property destruction, and emotional dysregulation.

A follow-up survey[16] of these specialized units identified high rates of ASD, communication impairment, and self-injury in the hospitalized population. Children with ASD made up 76% of the specialized inpatient population, totaling more than 1000 ASD cases per year. Most patients (88%) had a full-scale IQ of less than 75, and 25% exhibited self-injurious behaviors. The patients with ASD had particularly high rates of expressive communication impairment, with 27% classified as nonverbal (less than 10 words), 26% as limited verbal (primarily echolalia and scripting), and 45% as verbal (phrase speech). The median length of hospital stay was 30.5 days, and 13.8% of patients were readmitted within 1 year. All the specialized units used a combination of intervention approaches, including psychopharmacology, applied behavioral analysis, and individualized behavior plans. In addition to these core therapies, 63% of the units offered speech therapy, 50% offered occupational therapy, and 50% used family therapy.

Other countries, particularly England, Germany, and Canada, have also developed a small number of specialized units that serve the child ASD and ID populations. A survey of 136 hospitals with child psychiatry units in Germany found that 8% of these hospitals offered a specialized unit for the ASD and ID populations. Eighty-five percent of the respondents expressed a desire for a specialized unit.[17]

GENERAL CONSIDERATIONS FOR PSYCHIATRIC HOSPITAL CARE OF CHILDREN WITH ASD

The psychiatric hospital care of children with ASD requires consideration of the unique learning styles and needs of this population to guide the assessment and intervention process.

Assessment of Presenting Crisis Behaviors

The key initial treatment step is to accurately assess the issues underlying the presenting tip-of-the-iceberg crisis behaviors of patients with ASD.[18–20] This assessment process can be quite challenging, however, because typical psychiatric interview methods may not be reliable. Individuals with ASD, regardless of their language level, tend to have an impaired ability to reflect on and effectively communicate their internal experiences.[21] This challenge increases the risk that individuals with ASD will garner clinical attention for their unsafe behaviors, leaving the underlying cause of the behaviors underappreciated.

The Child and Caregiver Information Form, developed for use with the ASD and ID population, can provide a quick screen for etiologic domains of problem behaviors.[22] Successful treatment of problem behaviors in the ASD population is likely to increase if a broad differential diagnostic approach is used based on a multidisciplinary consideration of cause (**Table 1** and McGonigle and colleagues in this issue). At a general level, symptoms should be analyzed in terms of whether environmental (operant) conditions or intrinsic factors are responsible for the maintenance of the behavioral presentation. For example, one can consider whether the symptoms are best explained by environmental reinforcement, such as the removal of task demands

Table 1
Differential diagnosis of presenting problem behaviors in ASD/ID

Etiologic Domains	Examples of Potential Contributing Factors
Caregiver/community environment	• Environmental inconsistency • Inadvertent reinforcement of undesired behavior • Family dynamics/visitation schedules • Abuse/neglect • Individuation • Recent loss or change in the environment • Challenging social relationships (bullying) • Inappropriate school setting
Cognitive	• ID • Learning disability • Slow processing speed
Communication	• Absence of or inappropriate communication system • Use of communication system in only one setting
Genetic	• Fragile X, 22q11.2 deletion syndrome
Iatrogenic	• Polypharmacy • Sedation • Prompt dependence • Agitation from prolonged intensive behavioral management
Medical	• Pain • Seizures • Dental • Hearing • Vision • Pica • Constipation • Sleep • Allergies • Nutrition • Puberty • Brain injury
Psychopathologic	• Anxiety disorders, including posttraumatic stress disorder • Mood disorders • Attention-deficit/hyperactivity disorder, obsessive compulsive disorder • Psychosis or catatonia
Sensory-related	• Hypersensitivities or hyposensitivities to auditory, tactile, oral, visual, vestibular

Adapted from Siegel M. Psychopharmacology of autism spectrum disorder: evidence and practice. Child Adolesc Psychiatr Clin N Am 2012;21(4):962; with permission.

when a child strikes their educational aide, versus being neurobiologically mediated, such as aggression that arises when a severely anxious child experiences stimuli flooding. Inpatient admission also presents a unique opportunity to assess medical or environmental factors that may be contributing to a behavioral disturbance. For example, in the authors' experience, many children with ASD who were presumed to have a primary sleep disorder at home prove to sleep well in the hospital, suggesting an environmental cause. Additionally, **Case 1** provides an example of medical issues underlying a severe behavioral presentation in a nonverbal child with ASD.

CASE VIGNETTE 1: MEDICAL ISSUES IN CHILD WITH ASD

Sarah was a 12-year-old girl diagnosed with autistic disorder, ID, seizure disorder and mood disorder not otherwise specified. On admission to the neuropsychiatric special care (NSC) program at the Children's Hospital Colorado (formerly The Children's Hospital), Sarah was wearing a helmet because of her frequent head-banging behaviors. In addition, Sarah was nonverbal with no communication system, was not toilet trained, and frequently held her hand to her ear while making a very loud grunting/vibration noise and grimacing. Sarah routinely engaged in dangerous behaviors, including overturning furniture, aggression toward others, and self-injury (eg, head banging to the point of causing soft tissue damage, biting herself, and pinching and scratching herself). Several providers had told Sarah's parents that they needed to consider long-term institutionalization for Sarah because of the severity of her self-injurious behavior. Sarah had already been in a residential facility for 2.5 months, during which time she had refused to eat and lost 25 pounds. Sarah was then admitted to a general psychiatric unit where she had multiple staff and multiple psychotropic medications to manage her behaviors. Because of a lack of progress, Sarah was then transferred to the NSC program. On admission, Sarah's parents expressed concern that she had never seen a dentist. Previous institutions had not provided dental assessment because her providers and her insurance company determined that it was not medically necessary to see a dentist during a psychiatric hospitalization.

On admission to the NSC program, Sarah was immediately referred for a dental consultation within the hospital setting. Because of this consult, it was determined that Sarah had a black molar and a life-threatening jaw infection, which were quickly addressed. Almost immediately, Sarah's self-injurious behaviors disappeared; she no longer needed to wear a helmet, and she was calm and easily directed. Since Sarah's pain had been addressed, Milieu staff, including a speech therapist, were able to engage Sarah in learning to use simple signs to make requests, which she quickly learned and generalized to using with a variety of staff and with her father. Sarah's treatment team also began to question whether her hearing was impaired because of her insistence on seeking loud sounds. Sarah was then seen by the audiology department and found to be partially deaf in both ears. A hearing device was tried on Sarah, and she immediately responded by smiling and turning to look at her father when he called her name.

After 22 days, Sarah was discharged from the NSC program. She had learned to sit at a table and feed herself, give objects, and use some sign language to communicate her needs, as well as attend to individual work, social group, and toileting activities. After discharge, Sarah's father reported that Sarah had begun to say a few words and that he had learned that Sarah tends to have a calm disposition unless she is experiencing some kind of pain.

Psychiatric Comorbidity

Diagnosing comorbid psychopathology in children with ASD, particularly children with significant communication impairment, is a complex endeavor. Assessment must take into account whether a child's symptoms are typical of ASD, normal for developmental age, serve a specified adaptive function, and/or are modeled or reinforced in their environment, among other considerations. Children with ASD usually perform in an aberrant fashion on standard psychiatric diagnostic instruments that are designed for the neurotypical population, which can lead to the overidentification of comorbid psychiatric disorders. To address this, Leyfer and colleagues[2] (2006) modified the Kaufmann Schedule for Affective Disorders & Schizophrenia (K-SADS)[23] to account for symptoms typical of autism and for how psychiatric symptoms may present in children with ASD, producing the Autism Comorbidity Interview – Present and Lifetime Version (ACI-PL). The most frequently identified comorbid disorders were the following:

- Specific phobia (44%)
- OCD (37%)
- Attention-deficit/hyperactivity disorder (31%)

- Separation anxiety disorder (12%)
- Major depressive disorder (10%)

Clinicians should be wary of community-acquired comorbid psychiatric diagnoses as Mazefsky and colleagues[24] (2012) found that 60% of prior psychiatric diagnoses in a group of high-functioning adolescents with ASD were not supported by a psychiatric interview with the ACI-PL.

Verifying ASD Diagnosis and Cognitive Ability

A community diagnosis or the absence of a diagnosis of ASD or ID should not be taken at face value by the inpatient team. Verification of an ASD and/or ID diagnosis can allow for better-targeted interventions and recommendations for follow-up care in the community. A previously assigned diagnosis of ASD can be supported using a screening tool, such as the Social Communication Questionnaire.[25] A suspected new diagnosis of an ASD should be evaluated by the following:

1. Gathering developmental history about the patient from a primary caregiver using a standardized measure, such as the Autism Diagnostic Interview-Revised[26]
2. Using a standardized observational assessment of patients, such as the Autism Diagnostic Observation Schedule, Second Edition[27]

Using a standardized observational assessment administered by a trained evaluator can effectively tease out whether the patients' presenting social-communication difficulties are caused by ASD or another cause, such as an anxiety disorder or psychosis.

Obtaining reports from community providers regarding the patients' levels of intelligence, achievement, and adaptive functioning can assist in clarifying assessment issues and identifying appropriate interventions. Caregivers may tend to overestimate or underestimate the ability levels of their child with ASD because of the variability and inconsistent profile of adaptive and cognitive abilities common in this population.[28] Verbally based intelligence tests may not be reliable estimates of true problem-solving ability, particularly if the individual has coexisting language production, processing, or pragmatic impairments. In such cases, the Leiter International Performance Test, Revised[29] is a reliable cognitive screening tool for patients aged 2 to 21 years, and the brief IQ version takes approximately 30 minutes to administer.

Considering Communication

Receptive communication
Psychiatric settings typically rely on verbal instructions and intervention strategies. Individuals with ASD and ID, however, tend to process auditory information slowly. When they are provided with rapid or multiple pieces of verbal information, they can become agitated or unresponsive, which can be misinterpreted as resistant behaviors. The ASD population tends to think concretely, which can result in a tendency to follow directions in a literal manner.[30,31] The ASD population also has particular difficulty integrating and interpreting multiple pieces of social information (eg, tone of voice, facial expression, eye contact, and gestures).[32] This limitation can lead to the misperception of staff intentions and resultant agitation.

Strategies to increase comprehension include providing clear visual cues that have enough clarity for patients to understand and answer the following critical questions: What do I need to do? How much or how long do I do something? How do I know when I am finished? What do I do next? Strategies of visual clarity, schedules, and routines have empiric support for reducing behavior problems related to a lack of predictability and understanding of expectations.[33,34]

Expressive communication

Impaired ability to communicate even a basic need can cause great frustration for individuals with ASD and ID, and this can often be a sole cause for a resulting behavior problem. Helping patients communicate at any level can provide a prosocial means to getting their needs met.[35] It is recommended that psychiatric programs admitting ASD and ID populations routinely consult with speech language pathologists to identify and facilitate appropriate expressive communication strategies.

Hospital Environment

General psychiatric hospital environments are not typically adapted for the unique learning styles, needs, and abilities of the pediatric ASD or ID populations. Staff typically expect social and verbal initiations from patients, thus making it easy for individuals with ASD or ID to be ignored or forgotten in the regular daily operations of a busy psychiatric unit. Children with ASD may have abnormal responses to sensory stimuli, such as light, sound, touch and smells, that can make the hospital environment uncomfortable or even intolerable for some children. Minor modifications, such as dimming bright lights, choosing a patient room at a quieter end of the unit, providing noise-cancelling headphones, and access to fidget toys and quiet play spaces can significantly lessen agitation. It is recommended that psychiatric programs that admit the ASD/ID population routinely consult with occupational therapists to help assess and address sensory needs.

Structuring the environment can help individuals with ASD increase their attending behaviors and reduce challenging behaviors.[36] Environmental structure can range from providing picture schedules of routines, labeling containers, and designating routine locations with visual boundaries to having consistent routines paired with visual cues for activities and transitions. In addition to modifying the physical environment, patients' motivation can increase and challenging behaviors can be reduced when daily schedules alternate preferred and less-preferred activities.

Staff Training

General psychiatric hospital staff are not routinely trained to understand and effectively respond to this population.[37] Individuals with ASD or ID do not typically respond positively to the verbal strategies (eg, repetitive coaxing, verbal reassurance, or long explanations) or lengthy time-out procedures typically used with the neurotypical patient population. Additionally, not all staff prefer to work with the unique demands of patients with special needs. Training staff, including providing hands-on experience with the variety of functioning levels of patients with ASD and ID, is critical to reduce the risk for harm. Staff can be taught to alter their communication styles and management approaches, paying attention to their tone of voice and the complexity and amount of words used. Staff should be encouraged to allow patients extra time to process auditory information before repeating a direction or expecting a response. It is equally important for staff to resist the human urge to move in close to an individual who is in distress. Moving into close proximity or touching a distressed child with ASD or ID can be perceived as an intolerable sensory or emotional threat by the child. Backing away and giving patients time and space to process and deescalate is rarely the wrong thing to do.

EVIDENCE BASE FOR TREATMENT OF CHILDREN WITH ASD IN GENERAL PSYCHIATRIC HOSPITAL UNITS

There is very limited evidence for the treatment of children with ASD in general psychiatric hospital units. One retrospective case series described 29 adolescents with ASD hospitalized for acute behavioral regression in a French general adolescent psychiatry unit.[38] All the patients with ASD exhibited severe autistic symptoms and intellectual disability, two-thirds had no functional verbal language, and 48% had epilepsy. The average length of stay was 44 days, and a lower IQ was associated with longer length of stay.

The investigators assessed the cause of the disruptive behavior as adjustment disorder (24%), epilepsy (21%), inadequate outpatient therapy or educational services (21%), pain (10%), depression (7%) or catatonia (7%). The investigators concluded that adolescents with ASD need to be examined and treated with a multidisciplinary approach.

Some investigators have proposed concerns regarding the treatment of individuals with ASD or ID in general psychiatry units, such as exposing a vulnerable population to more able peers[39] or that staff typically lack training and experience in the assessment and treatment of comorbid psychopathology in this population.[40] One study reported that specialized units are perceived to provide a higher standard of care for individuals with ID.[41]

EVIDENCE BASE FOR SPECIALIZED PSYCHIATRIC HOSPITAL TREATMENT OF CHILDREN WITH ASD

There is a small and growing body of literature on the treatment effects of specialized inpatient psychiatry units for the adult and child populations with ASD and ID, although most studies have been retrospective and/or uncontrolled.

Adult Studies

A Finnish prospective study of 31 adult patients with borderline to mild ID and psychiatric symptoms described the treatment in a specialized psychiatric inpatient unit.[42] The treatment consisted of occupational therapy; group therapy; training in activities of daily living (ADL) skills; pharmacotherapy; financial guidance; psychoeducation; and other treatments, including music therapy; the average length of stay was almost 90 days. Psychotic symptoms were reduced on the Brief Psychiatric Rating Scale during hospitalization and at the 6-month follow-up, but nonpsychotic symptoms were reduced only at the follow-up.

A retrospective chart review of 13 adults with ASD admitted to a Canadian specialized inpatient psychiatry program showed an average length of stay of 295 days, 77% admitted with aggression, 15% with unmanageable behaviors, and 8% with self-harm/suicidality.[43] Another Canadian retrospective study of an adult specialized psychiatry unit with an average length of stay of 119 days compared outcomes for patients with mild ID with those with moderate/severe ID and found clinical improvement for both groups, but changes in standardized outcome measures did not reach significance.[44]

One descriptive study in the United Kingdom prospectively compared adults with ID admitted to a specialized psychiatric unit and a similar group admitted to a general psychiatric unit. The specialized unit cohort had a longer length of stay on average but demonstrated greater improvements on global measures of mental illness severity and was less likely to be discharged to a residential placement.[45]

Child and Adolescent Studies

The child literature begins with a report from 1972 describing an inpatient treatment program for children with autism or schizophrenia.[46] Children ranged from 4 to 12 years old, and the median length of stay was 2.25 years. The report describes the then-novel application of a daily routine of tasks and systematized reinforcement techniques, with positive results. Only 19 of the 57 children, however, were discharged to their homes.

In 1992, Barrett and colleagues[47] published an article describing a hospital program serving children with ASD or ID at Bradley Hospital. The program used applied behavioral analysis techniques and operant behavioral management principles in the context of a multidisciplinary intervention. The report stressed the importance of detecting and treating comorbid psychopathology. In a retrospective review of 50 serial admissions, they found an age range of 4 to 22 years, a 3:2 male/female ratio, 34% with ASD, and a wide range of comorbid axis I disorders. Characteristics of irritability and oppositionality were present in 80%.

In the United Kingdom, another case series identified 96 children with ID admitted to a specialized unit. The population was found to contain 2 subgroups: two-thirds had more severe disability and were admitted for neuropsychiatric management; one-third had problems more typical of mainstream psychiatry, but their ID was a barrier to mainstream psychiatric services.[44]

Gabriels and colleagues[48] provided the first support for the effectiveness of introducing a specialized inpatient psychiatric program for the treatment of children with ASD/ID. This retrospective chart review covered 2 eras of a psychiatric unit at the Children's Hospital Colorado. In the first era, children with ASD or ID were treated in a general child psychiatry unit, whereas, in the later era, a specialized unit was developed that included a step-down day treatment component. Twelve cases from the general treatment era and 26 cases from the specialized treatment era were compared. A dramatic decrease in the average length of stay from 45 days to 26 days and a decline in the recidivism rate (defined as readmission within 1 year) from 33% to 12% correlated with the change from the general to the specialized care era. In addition, the investigators found a significant decline from admission to discharge on the Aberrant Behavior Checklist[49]–Irritability and Hyperactivity subscales for children admitted to the specialized treatment program.

Recently, Siegel and colleagues[50] reported the first prospective study of a specialized inpatient psychiatry unit for children with ASD or ID using standardized outcome measures. Thirty-eight children, aged 5 to 18 years, were assessed by a consistent caregiver at admission, discharge, and 2 months after discharge on the Aberrant Behavior Checklist – Irritability (ABC-I) subscale. The ABC-I is a measure of behavioral functioning, evaluating aggression, self-injury, and tantrums, which has been shown to be valid and reliable for children with developmental disabilities. There was a substantial main treatment effect for time on the mean ABC-I score, which decreased from 27.3 (SD 7.4) at admission to 11.9 (SD 8.8) at discharge with slight regression to 14.8 (SD 9.3) at the 2-month follow-up (F $[2, 36]$ = 52.57, $P<.001$). Seventy-eight percent of the patients were rated as *much improved* or *very much improved* on a clinician-rated Clinical Global Impression - Improvement (CGI-I).

SPECIALIZED PSYCHIATRIC HOSPITAL TREATMENT MODELS
Model 1: Specialized Inpatient Treatment Unit

The Spring Harbor Hospital Developmental Disorders Unit (DDU) is a 12-bed specialized inpatient psychiatry program that performs assessment and treatment of comorbid psychopathology and acute behavioral disturbance in children with ASD and ID. Most patients present with unsafe behaviors toward themselves or others, and a small minority present with acute deterioration in functioning. Daily counts of physical aggression in the double digits and self-injurious behavior in the hundreds are common. The average length of stay is 42 days; 66% of the patients have ASD; greater than 80% have ID; and the average staffing ratio is 3 staff to 4 patients. Most children entering the program are at risk for out-of-home placement (residential or group home) and have been failed by multiple modes of prior treatment, including pharmacology, day treatment, in-home therapeutic services, and admission to general child psychiatry units. After treatment in the DDU, two-thirds of the children are discharged back to their home.

The treatment team consists of child psychiatry, pediatrics, behavioral psychology, a physician assistant, occupational therapy, speech and language pathology, social work, nursing, special education, and behavioral and educational technicians. Consultation from physical therapy, neurology, nutrition, genetics, and other specialties is available.

Treatment begins with an intensive multidisciplinary diagnostic assessment, typically aided by the removal of psychotropic medications. Details of the assessment approach are illustrated (**Case 2**). Treatment modalities include behavioral treatment based on principles of applied behavior analysis and positive reinforcement schema,

---

CASE VIGNETTE 2: CHILD BEHAVIORAL CHANGE OVER HOSPITAL STAY

Alana was a 7-year-old girl with autistic disorder, ID (mild to moderate), and significantly impaired communication (<50 words, primarily echolalia). Alana was admitted to the Spring Harbor Hospital Developmental Disorders Unit because of an acute increase in self-injurious behavior, tantrums, and aggression over the prior 2 months. Her mother estimated that Alana was emotionally dysregulated 50% of the time and engaged in self-injurious behavior more than 100 times a day, primarily by biting her hand or hitting her head with her hand. In the past, Alana had not responded to outpatient trials of clonazepam, risperidone, quetiapine, naltrexone, sertraline (5 mg/d), fluoxetine (5 mg/d), melatonin, and clonidine. Alana was awake for several hours nightly, which was highly disruptive for the family. Provision of 16 hours per week of in-home behavioral services, consisting of bachelor- and master-level providers, had been unsuccessful.

Initial multidisciplinary assessment revealed a tired girl who engaged in aggression and self-injury across home and school settings, primarily during tantrum episodes. Alana used a Picture Exchange Communication System (PECS)[51] at school but not outside that environment, and her independence with the system was minimal. Her tantrums were observed to occur primarily in relation to task demands or when denied preferred items. Alana's parents were assessed as being engaged with her treatment but were using minimal structure at home, relying mostly on psychopharmacology to attempt to decrease her aggression and self-injury.

Alana's initial hospital treatment focused on weaning her off clonidine and introducing a sleep routine, which included minimal attention during awake periods at night. This treatment resulted in much more consistent sleep, improved alertness, and reduced irritability. Target behaviors of emotional dysregulation, self-injury, and aggression were defined and operationalized and were tracked by the unit staff 24 hours a day. A positive behavioral support plan, utilizing a task:token economy, was developed to reinforce non-performance of target behaviors. PECS trials were initiated to assess and improve her communication efficiency.

Midway through her stay, it was determined that the token economy was too abstract for Alana, and she was changed to direct (ie, cause and effect) reinforcement of task completion. Alana was prepared for the end of each reinforcing activity by placing a visual countdown graphic next to her. A reduction in the frequency and duration of Alana's tantrums was obtained by creating a response routine whereby staff used a first/then visual card to reduce language demands and show her "first quiet voice," then (next activity). It was noted that her tantrums also occurred when she moved from one setting to another, which was addressed by using a preferred object as a transitional reinforcer, which was removed when tantrums occurred during the transition and returned when forward motion reinitiated.

Concurrently, a psychiatric assessment after a medication-free period diagnosed a generalized anxiety disorder, based on a consistent fear of elevators and entering group situations. Her anxiety decreased after initiation of sertraline at 25 mg/d (5 times the prior outpatient dosage). Occupational therapy and special education services provided Alana with sensory supports and academic task demands. Constipation was detected and treated with polyethylene glycol 3350 (MiraLax).

In the final phase of her hospitalization, Alana's parents were taught how to implement her behavioral plan, which included the first/then instruction card and other interventions described earlier. They then shadowed her staff and finally were coached by staff as they implemented the plan with Alana. Attendance by parents at a community PECS training course was facilitated by the unit social worker. Alana's parents were assisted in modifying the home environment to be more conducive to sleep and to implement visual supports. Alana's local school staff came into the hospital to observe the implementation of her behavior plan and supports. Outpatient services with a behavioral psychologist were arranged, and all supporting materials were transferred to her parents, the psychologist, and her school staff.

At discharge, Alana evidenced a 92% reduction in her daily number of self-injurious behaviors, a 66% decrease in her daily minutes of emotional dysregulation, and a 258% increase in her daily PECS exchanges (**Fig. 1**). After a 35-day hospital stay, Alana was discharged to her home.

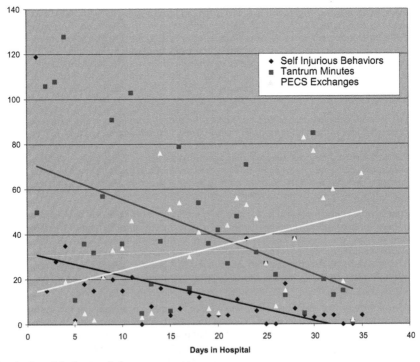

Fig. 1. Case 2 behavioral change over stay.

targeted psychopharmacology, treatment of acute medical issues, speech/language and occupational therapy, milieu therapy, special education, family therapy, and parent behavioral management training. Treatment is highly individualized; a verbal child with ASD and average IQ with explosive outbursts caused by social pragmatic deficits will receive treatment oriented toward cognitive flexibility and emotion regulation, whereas a more functionally challenged child with ASD with a high frequency of self-injurious behavior may receive high-density reinforcement of incompatible behaviors and in-depth occupational therapy support. The program runs its own 6-hour school day, and the school is often used as the laboratory to trial new interventions or behavioral plans.

The program seeks to address both the acute symptoms as well as the key underlying factors that contribute to the presentation of unsafe behavior. For example, identifying that an aggressive nonverbal child has no functional communication system might prompt treatment of the aggression with medication *and* training the child and family on the use of a visual picture communication system. The response to intervention is monitored by daily team analysis of behavioral data.

The benefits of family engagement in educational and behavioral interventions for children with ASD are well described.[52–54] Parental involvement has been deemed a critical component for reinforcing clinical treatments and promoting the generalization of learned skills to nonclinical environments. To this end, the primary caregivers of patients admitted to the program are offered the opportunity to participate in a 3-step behavior management training program where they are taught the child's individualized behavioral plan, shadow the staff running the plan, and ultimately run the plan themselves with staff supervision and coaching. Key community providers, such as local school staff and in-home therapeutic staff, are offered the same training. The goal of the program is to provide sustained improvement in behavioral functioning after discharge, and the readmission rate within 1 year is less than 10%.

Model 2: Specialized Inpatient Treatment with Integrated Step-down Model

The Neuropsychiatric Special Care (NSC) program at the Children's Hospital Colorado (previously, The Children's Hospital) is associated with the University of Colorado Anschutz Medical Center and is part of the Department of Psychiatry and Behavioral Sciences. In April 2004, this program was initiated to provide a specialized psychiatric continuum of care that includes both an inpatient unit and partial hospitalization program for patients aged 4 to 17 years diagnosed with ASD and/or ID who are in a state of crisis.[48] The partial hospitalization program component was developed to decrease lengthy inpatient stays and repeat admissions by allowing patients to leave the inpatient unit as soon their condition stabilizes, yet continue their involvement in the NSC program.

The objectives for designing this program were to develop a structured hospital environment with specialty-trained staff to address the following areas:

1. Decrease behavior problems related to patients' anxiety and limited social-communication skills so that the issues underlying presenting crisis behaviors could be better detected and addressed.
2. Decrease the need for high staffing ratios.
3. Increase the patients' involvement in a variety of milieu activities that simulate the community environment in order to assess the effects of interventions and promote generalization of skills into the community setting.
4. Increase caregiver sense of competence in understanding and managing patient behavior in order to decrease hospital recidivism rates.

Patients admitted to the NSC are assigned a core treatment team consisting of 3 professionals: a master-level clinician (family therapist/community coordinator), a psychologist (individual therapist/evaluator and behavior management coordinator), and a child psychiatrist (medical evaluation/management). Other staff include nursing and mental health counseling staff, creative arts therapists, occupational and speech therapists, and consulting medical specialty services as needed. At admission, the multidisciplinary staff conduct an evaluation process with the individual patient and their caregivers to identify intervention goals and plans. This process typically includes a milieu observational functional behavior assessment, an interactional assessment with patients and their caregivers, and a tip-of-the-iceberg assessment interview conducted by the psychologist with the patients' caregivers.

The structured setting and positive behavior intervention approach of the NSC program is based on cognitive behavioral and behavior learning theories. Specifically, NSC staff are trained on the TEACCH (Treatment and Education of Autistic and Related Communication Handicapped Children) model developed by the University of North Carolina, Chapel Hill, which capitalizes on the visual strengths of the ASD population to create highly structured and visually clear environments and routines. Intervention strategies are focused on taking a positive and proactive approach to managing challenging behaviors and teaching alternative functional behaviors.[34]

Caregiver education and involvement is a key component of the NSC program. Caregivers and community providers observe and interact with the patients in the therapeutic milieu with staff coaching and attend several different topic-specific weekly multifamily education-training groups. Direct-care staff maintain their competency with intervention methods by rotating participation in the multifamily groups, coleading weekly patient social groups with program therapists and psychologists, and daily consultation with psychologists about patients' behavior management plans.

IMPROVING CARE FOR ALL PSYCHIATRICALLY HOSPITALIZED INDIVIDUALS WITH ASD

Although most general psychiatry units do not have the resources to provide an extensive multidisciplinary team or a behavioral data collection and analysis system, the literature on specialized units suggests several avenues for improving the care of all individuals with ASD and ID admitted to psychiatric hospital units.

Clinical practice pathways have been shown to improve hospital care and outcomes for acute exacerbations of multiple chronic medical conditions, including congestive heart failure and ischemic heart disease.[50–56] The common components of these pathways include standardized evaluation components (draw a hemoglobin A1c and assess for foot health in all patients with diabetes), checklists to ensure the provision of proven treatment components (compression stockings and angiotensin-converting enzyme inhibitor for all admitted with congestive heart failure), and measurement of institutional benchmarks to track performance (readmission within 30 days and so forth). Psychiatric hospitals have been slower to adopt clinical practice pathways than medical hospitals, although acute psychiatric admission is commonly conceptualized as an exacerbation of a chronic illness.

Based on the extant literature and the authors' experience, the authors offer the following elements to consider as potential components of a clinical practice pathway for children or adults with ASD admitted to any psychiatric hospital unit (**Fig. 2**).

Other options for improving care include obtaining consultation from clinicians who specialize in the population or inserting a potentially critical treatment

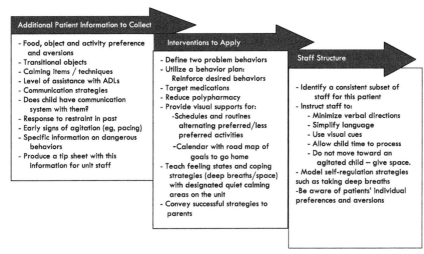

Additional Patient Information to Collect

- Food, object and activity preference and aversions
- Transitional objects
- Calming items / techniques
- Level of assistance with ADLs
- Communication strategies
- Does child have communication system with them?
- Response to restraint in past
- Early signs of agitation (eg, pacing)
- Specific information on dangerous behaviors
- Produce a tip sheet with this information for unit staff

Interventions to Apply

- Define two problem behaviors
- Utilize a behavior plan:
    Reinforce desired behaviors
- Target medications
- Reduce polypharmacy
- Provide visual supports for:
    -Schedules and routines alternating preferred/less preferred activities
    -Calendar with road map of goals to go home
- Teach feeling states and coping strategies (deep breaths/space) with designated quiet calming areas on the unit
- Convey successful strategies to parents

Staff Structure

- Identify a consistent subset of staff for this patient
- Instruct staff to:
    - Minimize verbal directions
    - Simplify language
    - Use visual cues
    - Allow child time to process
    - Do not move toward an agitated child – give space.
- Model self-regulation strategies such as taking deep breaths
- Be aware of patients' individual preferences and aversions

Fig. 2. Clinical practice pathway for psychiatrically hospitalized patients with ASD.

component, such as a functional behavioral analysis or a communication assessment, into the standard unit evaluation process when an individual with ASD or ID is admitted.

SUMMARY AND FUTURE DIRECTIONS

Children with ASD are psychiatrically hospitalized at disproportionately high rates, typically as a result of an acute decline in behavioral functioning. The core characteristics and presenting problems of the inpatient ASD population vary significantly from hospitalized neurotypical children because aggression and self-injurious behavior are the most common chief complaints. There is preliminary evidence that specialized inpatient treatment programs deliver positive behavioral outcomes for this population that endure 2 months after discharge. There are also multiple opportunities to improve ASD inpatient care.

As the number of children identified with ASD increases, the demand for inpatient psychiatric services is likely to continue to increase. This point elevates the importance of comparing the effectiveness of different treatment models and exploring the means of raising the standard of care for individuals with ASD in all hospital psychiatry settings.

ACKNOWLEDGMENTS

The authors thank Natalie Brim for her editorial suggestions.

REFERENCES

1. Bryson S, Smith I. Epidemiology of autism: prevalence, associated characteristics, and implications for research and service delivery. Ment Retard Dev Disabil Res Rev 1998;4(2):97–103.
2. Leyfer OT, Folstein SE, Bacalman S, et al. Comorbid psychiatric disorders in children with autism: interview development and rates of disorders. J Autism Dev Disord 2006;36:849–61.

3. Mandell DS. Psychiatric hospitalization among children with autism spectrum disorders. J Autism Dev Disord 2008;38(6):1059–65.

4. Croen LA, Najjar DV, Ray GT, et al. A comparison of health care utilization and costs of children with and without autism spectrum disorders in a large group model health plan. Pediatrics 2006;118(4):1203–11.

5. Harpaz-Rotem I, Leslie DL, Martin A, et al. Changes in child and adolescent inpatient psychiatric admission diagnoses between 1995 and 2000. Soc Psychiatry Psychiatr Epidemiol 2005;40(8):642–7.

6. Kalb LG, Stuart EA, Freedman B, et al. Psychiatric-related emergency department visits among children with an autism spectrum disorder. Pediatr Emerg Care 2012;28(12):1269–76.

7. Mandell DS, Xie M, Morales KH, et al. The interplay of outpatient services and psychiatric hospitalization among Medicaid-enrolled children with autism spectrum disorders. Arch Pediatr Adolesc Med 2012;166(1):68–73.

8. Autism and developmental disabilities monitoring network prevalence of autism spectrum disorders—autism and developmental disabilities monitoring network, 14 sites, United States, 2012. MMWR Surveill Summ 2012;61(3):1–19. Available at: www.cdc.gov/mmwr/pdf/ss/ss6103.pdf. Accessed April 1, 2012.

9. Ganz ML. The lifetime distribution of the incremental societal costs of autism. Arch Pediatr Adolesc Med 2007;161(4):343–9.

10. Shimbukuro TT, Grosse SD, Rice C. Medical expenditures for children with an autism spectrum disorder in a privately insured population. J Autism Dev Disord 2008;38(3):546–52.

11. American Psychiatric Association. Diagnostic and statistical manual of mental disorders. text rev. 4th edition. Washington, DC: American Psychiatric Association; 2000.

12. Reiss S, Levitan GW, Szyszko J. Emotional disturbance and mental retardation: diagnostic overshadowing. Am J Ment Defic 1982;86(6):567–74.

13. Wharff EA, Ginnis KB, Ross AM, et al. Predictors of psychiatric boarding in pediatric emergency department: implications for emergency care. Pediatr Emerg Care 2011;27(6):483–9.

14. Marrus N, Veenstra-Vander Weele J, Stigler K, et al. Training of general psychiatry residents and child and adolescent psychiatry fellows in autism and intellectual disability. Autism, in press.

15. Siegel M, Doyle K, Chemelski B, et al. Specialized inpatient psychiatry units for children with autism and developmental disorders: a United States survey. J Autism Dev Disord 2011;42(9):1863–9.

16. Siegel M, Teer O, Stein H, et al. Brief Report: Specialized inpatient psychiatry units for children with autism and developmental disorders - A follow-up survey. JADD, in submission.

17. Hennicke K. The care of mentally retarded children and adolescents with psychiatric disorders in hospitals for child and adolescent psychiatry and psychotherapy in Germany- results of a questionnaire survey. Z Kinder Jugendpsychiatr Psychother 2008;36(2):127–34 [in German].

18. Peeters T. (1995). The best treatment of behavior problems in autism is prevention. European Conference on Autism, University of Athens. Twachtman-Cullen D. and J.

19. Cox RD, Schopler E. Aggression and self-injurious behaviors in persons with autism–the TEACCH (treatment and education of autistic and related communications handicapped children) approach. Acta Paedopsychiatr 1993;56(2):85–90.

20. Gabriels RL. Adolescent transition to adulthood and vocational issues. In: Amaral D, Dawson G, Geschwind D, editors. Autism spectrum disorders. New York: Oxford University Press; 2011.
21. Mazefsky CA, Herrington J, Siegel M, et al. The role of emotion regulation in autism spectrum disorder. J Am Acad Child Adolesc Psychiatry 2013;52(7):679–88.
22. Gabriels RL. Understanding behavioral and emotional issues in autism. In: Gabriels RL, Hill DE, editors. Growing up with autism: working with school-age children and adolescents. New York: Guilford Press; 2007.
23. Kaufman J, Birmaher B, Brent D, et al. Schedule for affective disorders and schizophrenia for school-age children-present and lifetime version (K-SADS-PL): initial reliability and validity data. J Am Acad Child Adolesc Psychiatry 1997;36(7):980–8.
24. Mazefsky CA, Oswald DP, Day TN, et al. ASD, a psychiatric disorder, or both? Psychiatric diagnoses in adolescents with high-functioning ASD. J Clin Child Adolesc Psychol 2012;41(4):516–23.
25. Rutter M, Bailey A, Lord C. Social communication questionnaire. Los Angeles (CA): Western Psychological Services; 2003.
26. Lord C, Rutter M, LeCouteur A. Autism diagnostic interview-revised: a revised version of the diagnostic interview for caregivers of individuals with possible pervasive developmental disorders. J Autism Dev Disord 1994;24(5):659–85.
27. Lord C, Rutter M, DiLavore PC, et al. Autism diagnostic observation schedule 2nd edition manual. Los Angeles (CA): Western Psychological Services; 2012.
28. Bolte S, Poustka R. The relationship between general cognitive level and adaptive behavior domains in individuals with autism with and without co-morbid mental retardation. Child Psychiatry Hum Dev 2002;33(2):165–72.
29. Roid GH, Miller LJ. Leiter International Performance Scale-Revised (Leiter-R). Wood Dale (IL): Stoelting; 1997.
30. Twachtman-Cullen D, Twachtman-Reilly J. Communication and language issues in less-able school-aged children with autism. In: Gabriels RL, Hill DE, editors. Growing up with autism: working with school-age children and adolescents. New York: Guilford Press; 2007.
31. Twachtman-Cullen D. More able children with autism spectrum disorders. In: Wetherby AM, Prizant BM, editors. Autism spectrum disorders. Baltimore (MD): Paul H Brookes; 2000. p. 225–49.
32. Frith U. Autism: explaining the enigma. Proceedings. United Kingdom: Blackwell Publishing; 2003.
33. Mesibov GB, Browder DM, Kirkland C. Using individualized schedules as a component of positive behavioral support for students with developmental disabilities. J Positive Behavioral Interventions 2002;4:73–9.
34. Mesibov GB, Shea V. The TEACCH program in the era of evidence-based practice. J Autism Dev Disord 2010;40(5):570–9.
35. O'Reilly M, Sigafoos J, Lancioni G, et al. An examination of the effects of a classroom activity schedule on levels of self-injury and engagement for a child with severe autism. J Autism Dev Disord 2005;35(3):305–11.
36. Rogers SJ. Intervention for young children with autism: from research to practice. Infants and Young Children 1999;12(2):1–16.
37. Heidgerken AD, Geffken G, Modi A, et al. A survey of autism knowledge in a healthcare setting. J Autism Dev Disord 2005;35(3):323–30.
38. Périsse D, Amiet C, Consoli A, et al. Risk factors of acute behavioral regression in psychiatrically hospitalized adolescents with autism. J Can Acad Child Adolesc Psychiatry 2010;19(2):100–8.

39. Kwok HW. Development of a specialized psychiatric service for people with learning disabilities and mental health problems: report of a project from Kwai Chung Hospital, Hong Kong. British J Learning Disabilities 2001;29(1):22–5.

40. Bouras N, Holt G. Community mental health services for adults with learning disabilities. In: Thornicroft G, Szmukler G, editors. Textbook of community psychiatry. London: Oxford University Press; 2001. p. 397–407.

41. Lennox N, Chaplin R. The psychiatric care of people with intellectual disabilities: perceptions of trainee psychiatrists and psychiatric medical officers. Aust N Z J Psychiatry 1995;29(4):632–7.

42. Raitasuo S, Taiminen T, Salokangas RK. Inpatient care and its outcome in a specialist psychiatric unit for people with intellectual disability: a prospective study. J Intellect Disabil Res 1999;43(2):119–27.

43. Palucka AM, Lunsky Y. Review of inpatient admissions of individuals with autism spectrum disorders to a specialized dual diagnosis program. J Dev Disabil 2007;13(1):206–9.

44. Smith P, Berney TP. Psychiatric inpatient units for children and adolescents with intellectual disability. J Intellect Disabil Res 2006;50(8):608–14.

45. Xenitidis K, Gratsa A, Bouras N, et al. Psychiatric inpatient care for adults with intellectual disabilities: generic or specialist units? J Intellect Disabil Res 2004; 48(1):11–8.

46. Treffert DA, McAndrew JB, Dreifuerst P. An inpatient treatment program and outcome for 57 autistic and schizophrenic children. J Autism Child Schizophr 1973;3(2):138–53.

47. Barrett RP, Walters AS, Mercurio AF. Mental retardation and psychiatric disorders. In: Van Hasselt VB, Kolko DJ, editors. Inpatient behavior therapy for children and adolescents. New York: Springer; 1992.

48. Gabriels RL, Agnew JA, Beresford C, et al. Improving psychiatric hospital care for pediatric patients with autism spectrum disorders and intellectual disabilities. Autism Res Treat 2012. http://dx.doi.org/10.1155/2012/685053.

49. Aman M, Singh N, Stewart A, et al. The aberrant behavior checklist: a behavior rating scale for the assessment of treatment effects. Am J Ment Defic 1985;89: 485–91.

50. Siegel M, Milligan B, Chemelski B, et al. Specialized inpatient psychiatric treatment for serious behavioral disturbance in autism and intellectual disability, submitted, 2013.

51. Bondy A, Frost L. The picture exchange communication system. Behav Modif 2001;25(5):725–44.

52. Benson P, Karlof KL, Siperstein GN. Maternal involvement in the education of young children with autism spectrum disorders. Autism 2008;12(1):47–63.

53. Moes DR, Frea WD. Contextualized behavior support in early intervention for children with autism and their families. J Autism Dev Disord 2002;32(6):519–33.

54. Scahill L, McDougle CJ, Aman MG, et al. Effects of risperidone and parent training on adaptive functioning in children with pervasive developmental disorders and serious behavioral problems. J Am Acad Child Adolesc Psychiatry 2012;51(2):136–46.

55. Ranjan A, Tarigopula L, Srivastava RK, et al. Effectiveness of the clinical pathway in the management of congestive heart failure. South Med J 2003; 96(7):661–3.

56. Aziz EF, Javed F, Pulimi A, et al. Implementing a pathway for the management of acute coronary syndrome leads to improved compliance with guidelines and a decrease in angina symptoms. J Healthc Qual 2012;34(4):5–14.

The Family Context of Autism Spectrum Disorders

Influence on the Behavioral Phenotype and Quality of Life

Leann E. Smith, PhD[a], Jan S. Greenberg, PhD[b],
Marsha R. Mailick, PhD[a],*

KEYWORDS

- Autism spectrum disorders • Family • Stress • Psychoeducation
- Expressed emotion

KEY POINTS

- A growing body of research has documented the high level of stress that parents of individuals with ASD experience and the subsequent impact of stress on parental well-being.
- Few have studied the reverse direction of effects: the influence of the family environment on the behavioral phenotype of ASD.
- Reducing levels of criticism and increasing levels of warmth in the family may help prevent the development and escalation of severe behavior problems in children, adolescents, and adults with ASD.
- *Transitioning Together*, an 8-week, multifamily group psychoeducation program, was developed to improve the family environment and meet the needs of families of individuals with ASD for education and support.
- Future research is needed to identify other best practice models in working with families of persons with ASD.

INTRODUCTION

Parents of children with autism spectrum disorder (ASDs) experience high levels of stress as caregivers.[1,2] The challenging behaviors presented by many children on the spectrum is one of the most significant sources of stress for families.[3–5] These behavior problems can continue into adulthood, creating barriers for adult

The authors have nothing to disclose.
[a] Waisman Center, University of Wisconsin-Madison, 1500 Highland Avenue, Madison, WI 53705, USA; [b] School of Social Work, Waisman Center, University of Wisconsin-Madison, 1500 Highland Avenue, Madison, WI 53705, USA
* Corresponding author.
E-mail address: Mailick@Waisman.Wisc.Edu

independence and community involvement.[6] Although there is evidence of some abatement of autism symptoms and behavior problems over time,[7,8] ASD is a lifelong disability that presents multiple challenges for families at each stage of the life course.

Our research has documented significant levels of stress associated with parenting a child with ASD during adolescence and adulthood and the impact of this stress on maternal health and well-being. In a daily diary study of mothers over an 8-day period[9] we found that mothers of adolescents and adults with ASD were three times more likely to experience a stressful event on a given day than mothers of children without disabilities. These stressful daily experiences had a negative impact on mothers' emotional and physical well-being. Our research has demonstrated that mothers of adults with ASD have significantly more physical health symptoms, such as joint pain, fatigue, headaches, and gastrointestinal problems, than mothers of adults without disabilities.[10] Furthermore, we examined differences in cortisol expression between mothers of adolescents and adults with ASD and mothers of similar-aged children without disabilities and found that mothers of individuals with ASD had significantly hypoactivated cortisol levels.[11] This pattern of a chronic stress response is similar to what has been found in individuals with caregiver burnout and posttraumatic stress disorder. The history of behavior problems in the adolescents and adults in our sample significantly moderated the association between daily stress and cortisol level, with mothers of a son or daughter with clinically significant levels of behavior problems over the previous 5-year period having a blunted cortisol response in the face of daily stress, reflecting a greater hypoactivation of cortisol and a chronic stress response. These findings clearly highlight the significant risks to parental emotional and physical well-being associated with raising a child with ASD.

Perhaps in reaction to the history of blaming families of children with autism, researchers have been reluctant to examine the reverse direction of effects (ie, the influence of the family environment on the behavioral phenotype of autism). Given the centrality of the family in helping maximize the quality of life of persons with autism, there is a need to identify those characteristics of the family environment that are associated with the abatement versus escalation of behavior problems over time. In this article, we report the findings from our research examining the bidirectional influence between the family environment and the behavioral phenotype of autism, and describe a newly developed family psychoeducation program to reduce family stress, reduce behavior problems, and improve the quality of life of adolescents with autism and their families.

EXPRESSED EMOTION AND BEHAVIORAL DIFFICULTIES

To identify characteristics of the family environment that may influence the course of a child's disability, researchers studying persons with psychiatric disorders have paid considerable attention to the phenomenon of expressed emotion (EE).[12] EE was originally conceptualized in terms of five dimensions of the family environment (criticism, hostility, emotional overinvolvement, warmth, and positive remarks), which were initially assessed by the administration of the Camberwell Family Interview.[13] In early studies of the effects of EE on relapse rates in adults with schizophrenia, Brown and colleagues[14] found that it was the criticism dimension that was the crucial variable in predicting symptomatic relapse, with emotional overinvolvement independently predicting relapse in a small number of cases. Consequently, subsequent studies focused on these two dimensions in operationalizing high EE. Since this initial work, a large number of studies have implicated EE in predicting symptom exacerbations across a broad range of mental health disorders and medical conditions, including schizophrenia, mood disorders, eating disorders, Alzheimer disease, asthma, diabetes, and Parkinson disease.[15,16]

More recently the construct of EE has been explored in families of typically developing children and adolescents[17,18] and families of individuals with intellectual and developmental disabilities (IDD).[19–22] In families of typically developing children, higher levels of parental criticism have been associated with more problematic child behaviors at multiple points in the life course.[17,18,21,23] Parental criticism has likewise been linked with behavior problems in children and adolescents with IDD.[4,20] In a review of studies of EE in families of children with IDD, Hastings and Lloyd[24] argued that although the challenges associated with caring for an individual with IDD may create a family context where some level of EE is to be expected, the presence of high EE in families may exacerbate or maintain behavior problems and that research is needed to understand how to most effectively intervene to help these families.

FAMILIES OF ADOLESCENTS AND ADULTS WITH AUTISM

Our longitudinal research, spanning a 13-year period in a large cohort of families of adolescents and adults with ASD, has investigated separate dimensions of EE to identify characteristics of the family environment that influence the behavioral phenotype of adolescents and adults with autism. However, rather than focusing only on the negative dimensions of the family environment, our approach has been to broaden the focus to also include positive dimensions of family life, such as warmth and positive remarks that may promote positive behavior in the son or daughter with ASD and such dimensions as high levels of criticism that may result in an escalation of behavior problems or worsening of symptoms. The data for the analyses reported here come from a larger study of 406 families of adolescents and adults with an ASD who have been followed since 1999.[25,26] The families met three criteria when initially recruited: (1) the son or daughter was age 10 or older; (2) he or she had received a diagnosis on the autism spectrum from a medical, psychological, or educational professional, as reported by the parents; and (3) administration of the Autism Diagnostic Interview–Revised (ADI-R)[27] confirmed the parental report of an ASD.

Mothers were interviewed in their homes and also completed standardized self-administered measures. At the beginning of the study, the mothers ranged in age from 32 to 81 and their sons and daughters ranged from 10 to 52. Almost 65% of the individuals with ASD lived at home when the study began, and 49% still live in the family home 13 years later. Of the individuals with autism, 73% were male and 70% had an intellectual disability diagnosis.

As part of the interviews, we administered the Five Minute Speech Sample (FMSS),[28] which was based on the Camberwell Family Interview, to measure the family environment. For the FMSS, the mother is asked to speak for 5 minutes to describe her relationship with the son or daughter with autism and to express her thoughts and feelings about this individual. The FMSS is coded both with respect to verbal content and vocal tone, and measures of maternal criticism, emotional overinvolvement, warmth, and positive remarks can be derived from this coding based on standard coding procedures.[28] Hostility cannot be separately coded using the FMSS because of its high correlation with criticism.

Briefly, respondents are rated as "high" on criticism if they describe their relationship with their son or daughter in negative terms, or if they make one or more criticisms about their son or daughter during the course of the 5-minute speech sample.

The following transcript, which represents a composite case, provides an example of how a parent classified as high in criticism speaks about the relationship with her child with autism:

> David is a very wonderful, kind-hearted boy. He's motivated to do what's expected of him and tries very hard. But he has a lot of limitations. He has no peer relationships. He is very challenging because he needs a lot of input from us. He's dependent on us to provide his recreation all the time and it gets really difficult. One of the biggest problems is to structure his time. I've had to deal with that throughout his life. He may enjoy doing something 1 day and the next absolutely refuse to do it so it is really hard to find things that motivate him. The other difficulty is that he wants many, many material items. His appetite for material items is insatiable and it is constantly a battle to get him to understand that we are not a bottomless money pit.

Emotional overinvolvement occurs when the family member either expresses excessive self-sacrificing or overprotective feelings toward the son or daughter with autism. Because autism requires that many parents make personal sacrifices to care for their child and may need to protect their child from being harmed by self or others, a rating of emotional overinvolvement requires that the behavior be "excessive." The following composite transcript captures the meaning of emotional overinvolvement in autism.

> Susie is the biggest challenge of my life. She can make us cry in a heartbeat and she can make us laugh in a heartbeat. It's always about her; our life revolves around whatever works for Susie. Everything that affects her affects us. I know my life would be entirely different without her. We don't go to restaurants; we don't go to movies; we don't do family activities, and sometimes my sadness is for the other kids that they never experienced what a lot of their friends have. I care a lot about her, maybe too much, but I feel like I need to protect her to the maximum. I often times wonder how much of my identity is wrapped up in her. Where is the line? Where does Susie end and I begin?

Warmth ratings are based on (1) tone of voice; (2) spontaneity of expression of sympathy, concern, or empathy; and (3) expression of interest in the child with autism. The following transcript represents a composite case of how a mother classified as high in warmth speaks about her child.

> My son Steve is a wonderful, loving upbeat beautiful man and I am very, very proud of him. We live out here on our farm. Steve gets up every day faithfully and works diligently in providing care for the animals and it has helped him. He just seems to feel more important because he knows that these animals depend upon him and care. Right now we are in the process of canning and Steve is learning horticulture. We are about to have our first grandchild and Steve is going to be an uncle for the very first time and he's excited about that. He got to help his brother participate in the naming of the baby.

Positive remarks reflect the number of positive statements the respondents expresses about her child during the FMSS. The following transcript, which represents a composite case, provides an example of a mother high on positive remarks.

> He's so amazing. He's very kind hearted and he's honest. And his randomness is such a unique personality. People really just love him. He tries hard to understand what other people are feeling and doing. He doesn't like to complain about feeling bad or being sick, so if he does you know it's really bad. He doesn't mind helping usually and he loves to learn. Since he started Special Olympics, he's just blossomed. He can run now; he took third place in one of his meets and it was unbelievable because he ran like no one was looking at him.

To investigate the association between the family environment and the behavioral phenotype of ASD, we administer the Problem Behavior subscale of the Scales of Independent Behavior–Revised (SIB-R)[29] and the ADI-R[27] to the families in our study. These measures were administered repeatedly (at four points of data collection over a 7-year period) to measure change. Standardized algorithms[29] are used to translate SIB-R frequency and severity ratings into three subscales scores: (1) Internalized Maladaptive Behavior, (2) Asocial Maladaptive Behavior, and (3) Externalized Maladaptive Behavior. The ADI-R is a standardized investigator-based interview conducted with a primary caregiver (in our case, with the mother of the individual with autism). Based on the items in the diagnostic algorithm[8] the ADI-R yields ratings for the three primary symptom clusters used in the diagnosis of autism: (1) repetitive behaviors and restricted interests, (2) impairment in reciprocal social interaction, and (3) impairments in communication. The repeated measures of the FMSS (to assess the family environment), SIB-R (to assess behavior problems), and ADI-R (to assess autism symptoms) make it possible to examine how aspects of the family environment predict change in the behavior problems and autism symptoms of the son or daughter, and whether the reverse direction of effects (from the child's behavior problems and autism symptoms to the family environment) is also evident.

Although we find evidence of bidirectional influences between the family environment factors and child functioning, the direction of effects seems to be primarily from the family to the child. In our first study investigating 149 mothers coresiding with an adolescent or adult with autism, we found that family environments marked by high levels of criticism predicted increases in the severity of internalizing and asocial behavior problems and in repetitive behaviors and restricted interests over the 18-month period, controlling for prior levels of behavior problems and autism symptoms.[30] Furthermore, in a follow-up analysis of the same sample, we examined growth curve trajectories of criticism and behavior problems over a 7-year period. We found that increases in criticism over the 7 years were associated with higher levels of behavior problems at the final time point, whereas change in behavior problems did not significantly predict final levels of criticism.[31]

We subsequently conducted a parallel longitudinal study of 122 mothers of children (ages 6–8) and adolescents (ages 12–21) with fragile X syndrome (FXS).[32] In this study, we found similar relationships between high levels of maternal criticism and an increase in internalizing, externalizing, and total problems as measured by the Child (or Adult) Behavior Checklist (A/CBCL),[33,34] although the patterns were somewhat different in families of children and families of adolescents. Higher levels of maternal criticism were related to a subsequent increase in externalizing and total problems in the children with FXS, and to an increase in internalizing behavior problems, externalizing, and total behavior problems in the adolescents with FXS. Thus, one consistent finding of our research on families of persons with developmental disabilities is the pervasive negative effect that a high level of parental criticism has on child behavior.

We also found evidence that high levels of maternal warmth and positive remarks are associated with reductions in autism symptoms in our longitudinal research on families of adolescents and adults with autism. High levels of maternal warmth and positive remarks were related to declining levels of repetitive behaviors and restricted interests, as measured by the ADI-R 18 months later.[35] This direction of effects was similar to the patterns we found between criticism and behavior problems summarized previously (ie, from warmth and positive remarks to behavior problems). We did not find evidence for the reverse direction of effects. Thus, we did not find that prior levels of behavior problems or autism symptoms affected levels of maternal warmth or positive remarks 18 months later. In our parallel longitudinal study of families of children and adolescents with FXS, we similarly found that high levels of maternal warmth were related to declining levels of total behavior problems and to declining levels of externalizing problems (as measured by the A/CBCL) for children with FXS (but maternal warmth did not have a significant effect on the behavior of adolescents).

In a related study of a subset of the families in our longitudinal research on autism, we examined how exiting high school affected the behavior of adolescents with autism and also the relationship of the adolescent with his or her mother.[36,37] For those adolescents with autism who did not have a comorbid intellectual disability, maternal warmth was found to decline after the son or daughter left high school, although this was not the case for mothers of adolescents with intellectual disabilities. This finding suggested that although behavior problems did not directly affect maternal warmth, changes in the daily life of the young adult with autism (ie, exiting high school) did have an influence on maternal warmth.

Taken together, our findings suggest that reducing high levels of criticism (or maintaining low levels of criticism) and increasing parental warmth may prevent an escalation of behavior problems and autism symptoms. Thus, the family environment is an important target for intervention not only to reduce family distress but also to improve functioning for the child, adolescent, or adult with ASD. From a family systems perspective, transition periods, such as adolescence, may be particularly effective times for interventions, given that reorganizations in the family system are taking place during this stage of life.[38] Furthermore, the findings reported previously based on Taylor and Seltzer's research[37] suggest that maternal warmth may be disrupted by transitions in the life of the son or daughter with autism, and thus adolescence may be an ideal time to intervene at the family level, which has led our group to develop a family psychoeducational program known as *Transitioning Together*.

The Transitioning Together Program

Multifamily group psychoeducation is a well-validated intervention approach for families of individuals with psychiatric conditions.[39–41] Psychoeducation interventions for mental health conditions typically provide families with information about what is known about the cause, course, and outcome of the condition; effective interventions and treatments; community supports and resources; how the family is affected; behavior management; and vocational and residential planning.[42] The effectiveness of psychoeducation interventions in improving the overall family environment and reducing behavior problems and symptoms in individuals with mental health conditions has been demonstrated in multiple studies of conditions, such as schizophrenia[43,44] and mood disorders.[45–47] However, such programs had yet to be developed and evaluated for families of children with autism. Our primary goal in developing *Transitioning Together* was to determine whether a psychoeducational group intervention would reduce family stress and behavior problems, and improve the quality of life of persons with autism and their families.

Consistent with a multifamily psychoeducation model, the *Transitioning Together* program[48] has two stages of intervention: two individual-family joining sessions and eight multifamily group sessions. The joining sessions allow the family to meet with the intervention staff before the group meetings to develop rapport and clarify family goals. After completing the joining sessions, families attend eight weekly group sessions. Group sessions involve education on a variety of topics relevant to ASD and guided practice with problem-solving for individual family problems. The topics and goals for each session are presented in **Table 1**.

Table 1
Summary of intervention session topics

Session	Topic	Goals
Group Meeting 1	Autism in Adulthood	Meet other families [a]Learn about developmental course of ASD
Group Meeting 2	Transition Planning	[a]Learn about education, occupational, residential, service system, and health transition
Group Meeting 3	Problem Solving	Learn and practice problem-solving method
Group Meeting 4	Family Topics	[a]Learn about how family environment impacts behaviors
Group Meeting 5	Addressing Risks to Adult Independence	[a]Learn strategies for behavior management during late adolescence and early adulthood [a]Discuss advocacy strategies when behaviors are misunderstood by community
Group Meeting 6	Community Involvement	[a]Finding community activities and social opportunities Discuss safety concerns for adults with ASD
Group Meeting 7	Risks to Health	[a]Learn about risks to parental health and well-being
Group Meeting 8	Legal Issues	Receive information on long-term planning: guardianship, wills, trusts, etc

[a] Indicates content based on published findings of our research group.
From Smith LE, Greenberg JS, Mailick MR. Adults with autism: outcomes, family effects, and the multifamily group psychoeducation model. Curr Psychiatry Rep 2012;14:735; with permission.

Sessions last approximately 1.5 hours each. Sessions begin with 15 minutes of socializing, followed by 30 minutes of presentation on a topic and 45 minutes of discussion and problem-solving. For each problem-solving activity, one family's problem is chosen by the group. Next, the group works together to select strategies that the family can implement to address that problem. The family is able to share updates on strategy implementation the following week. This process provides an opportunity to gain from the vast experiences of the multiple participating families and to focus on addressing problems in a constructive, noncritical way. In addition to group problem-solving, families also receive individualized resources and referrals based on needs expressed during sessions (eg, mental health providers, summer camps). At the same time and location (but in a different room) as the parent group sessions, the adolescents with ASD participate in a social group, which involves a variety of games and learning activities on such topics as sharing interests, setting goals, social problem solving, and party planning.

Our initial pilot evaluation of the *Transitioning Together* program included 10 families of adolescents with ASD (aged 15–18 years; M = 16.2; SD = 1.1). Even with this very small sample, we found significant positive changes from preintervention to postintervention in parents' understanding of their child's disability and of the service system.[48] There were also significant improvements in the parent-child relationship domain. Importantly, parents were rated (by an independent blind rater) as having higher levels of warmth toward their son or daughter, based on coding of the FMSS. Furthermore, after the intervention, parents were more likely to report being happy or proud of their child. Although we did not find significant changes in autism symptoms or in parental report of stress in this small pilot sample, parents increased in their ability to predict when their child would have a behavior problem from preintervention to postintervention.[48]

Currently we are evaluating a refined version of the *Transitioning Together* program with a highly homogenous group of families. Our pilot study was comprised of adolescents with a wide range of verbal and intellectual abilities, including individuals with intellectual disability along with individuals with IQs in the gifted range. The inclusion criteria for our new evaluation study are that participating families have adolescents between the ages of 14 and 17 years who are verbal (speak using complex sentences) and who particulate in general education settings at least 50% of the time. We believe that by creating homogenous groups, parent and teenage sessions will be more focused and beneficial for families, with even larger observable gains in quality of life. In this current study, we have increased the sample to include 40 families and broadened the range of outcome measures to include parental well-being, burden, and daily stress (including a measure of salivary cortisol) and adolescent social and recreational activities, friendships, and adaptive behavior.

COMPOSITE CASE OF A FAMILY WHO COMPLETED THE *TRANSITIONING TOGETHER* PROGRAM

CASE: COMPOSITE CASE OF FAMILY IN TRANSITIONING TOGETHER PROGRAM

Becky is a single mother of a 16-year-old son, John, who has ASD. John is a junior in a large public high school and he has two older sisters who no longer live at home. He enjoys videogames and is fascinated with Chinese culture. Although John has above average intelligence (Wechsler Full Scale IQ of 125) and does well in many academic subjects, he has significant delays in adaptive behavior (eg, difficulties with hygiene; Vineland Standard Score of 67). At time of entry into the *Transitioning Together* study, John had total scores in the clinical range on measures of behavior problems and psychopathology (SIB-R and CBCL) and was taking medication for anxiety. He exhibited a range of challenging behaviors including being hurtful to himself, hurtful to others, disruptive, withdrawn, uncooperative, and having repetitive habits.

Before beginning the intervention, Becky reported a high level of stress on the Perceived StressScale[49] and her responses during the FMSS indicated a high level of EE:

My relationship with John, well, I wish it was better. I wish for more. I try to talk to him about important things and I can't have a conversation, a real conversation with him. I hope that as he grows older that will change.

After completion of the *Transitioning Together* program, the family displayed positive changes that were consistent with the program's goals of reducing family stress and improving quality of life. For example, there was an improvement in the parent-child relationship, which was evidenced in the FMSS taken during the exit interview:

As far as my relationship with John, he has a great sense of humor, and he loves to have intellectual conversation with me. He shares science facts with me and we joke around a lot. His sisters think he's funny too. I really enjoy that aspect of our relationship.

Becky also reported lower levels of stress after the intervention, although her overall stress levels were still elevated. During the exit interview Becky reflected on her experience in the program, saying:

I think probably what was most useful to me was just hearing from other families, hearing about the challenges they have with their teens too and getting ideas for handling issues. At times with my kids I've felt very isolated and alone. Hearing other families talk about having the same types of experiences was really validating. And it was nice to toss out my ideas that could maybe help others. The group reminded me that some of these things are just a part of autism.

Participating in *Transitioning Together* also had a positive impact on John. Over the course of the eight group sessions he became increasingly more engaged in group interactions, as rated by the intervention staff. There also was noticeable improvement in John's challenging behaviors. Based on an adapted, daily version of the SIB-R, John's level of daily behavior problems dropped by 12% after the intervention. Also, although his CBCL total score was still within the clinical range after the intervention, the general trend was one of improvement. On one subscale (conduct disorders), John's scores were in the borderline clinical range before the intervention but were in the normal range after the intervention. Unfortunately, John did not show significant change in autism symptoms (as measured by the Social Responsivity Scale).[50] The lack of change in autism symptoms and the continued high levels of many behavior problems are consistent with our prior findings and highlight the pervasive nature of ASD and the likely need for continuing, intensive interventions for individuals and their families.

During the exit interview, John indicated that he learned better ways to do things like organizing and planning, which he thinks will help him in the future. He particularly appreciated getting to meet other teenagers his age.

The thing I liked best was probably just meeting the other guys. We were all juniors so it was neat to meet other people like me going through the same types of things at school. We would share about our weeks. One person might make a joke and then someone else would make a follow up on it and that was just great. Of course I would usually be the one making the jokes!

In addition to providing humor for the group, John believed that he contributed good ideas: "I was a good observer and listener, and when I did say something it was a good point." Reflecting on insights he had over the course of the group John also said, "Mostly I've been thinking about how far I've come since I was a kid. And I think I've figured out that my brain works differently from most people. That's what I've been thinking."

SUMMARY AND FUTURE DIRECTIONS

In other studies based on our ongoing research, we have reported poor outcomes for adults with autism in important areas that determine their quality of life. For example, we have shown that adaptive behavior in adults with autism lags behind their cognitive capacities,[51] that high school exit marks a time of increased vulnerability with respect to behavior problems and autism symptoms,[36] that friendships are scarce in adulthood and social participation is not frequent,[52] that vocational outcomes are poor and tend to decline over time,[53] and that few live independently.[54]

In this article reviews our research that has shown that the quality of the relationship between parents and the adolescent or adult with autism can be an important factor shaping trajectories of behavioral functioning in the son or daughter. Our findings are completely consistent with the large body of research summarized previously in this paper showing that the family environment, as indexed by EE, can have a significant effect on the functioning of individuals with mental health problems; developmental problems; and physical illnesses as diverse as asthma, attention-deficit/hyperactivity disorder, Parkinson disease, and schizophrenia, and now autism and FXS. As such, criticism and warmth might best be conceptualized as powerful aspects of intimate relationships that can significantly affect the manifestation and severity of symptoms.

There currently is significant interest in bullying as experienced by children and adolescents with autism[55–57] and the effect of bullying on their mental health. Perhaps bullying is a particularly intense form of criticism and may be a factor that affects the gap between the cognitive capacities and adaptive behavior of those who have autism, and the persistence of their behavior problems and autism symptoms. Furthermore, it would be valuable to ascertain the extent to which criticism in the relationships between adults with autism and other key figures in their lives, such as employers or coworkers, is also implicated in the poor quality of life that such adults typically experience.

Transitioning Together is a promising intervention that may have the effect of reducing family distress during the time when the son or daughter with autism is transitioning to adulthood. Given the centrality of the family in the lives of adults with autism, and their continued need for support, the positivity of their relationships with their parents and siblings may be particularly important for behavioral regulation, social integration, and quality of life. Because of the rapid increase of autism diagnoses since the 1990s, more children than ever before are entering adulthood with an autism diagnosis. Despite a pressing need for research and interventions during this transition period, there currently are very few empirically validated programs for adolescents with autism or their families. Multifamily group psychoeducation, such as *Transitioning Together*, is one promising approach to address these needs and potentially ameliorate risks for individuals with adults and their families during the transition to adulthood and beyond.

ACKNOWLEDGMENTS

This research is supported by grants from the National Institute on Aging (R01 AG08768, M.R. Mailick, PI); the National Institute on Child Health and Human Development (P30 HD03352, M.R. Mailick, PI); and Autism Speaks (7523, L. Smith, PI). The authors gratefully acknowledge support from UW-Madison's Clinical and Translational Science Award Program for community intervention research (supported in part by grant U21 RR025011); the Autism Society of Southeastern Wisconsin; the Graduate School; and the Waisman Center at the University of Wisconsin-Madison.

REFERENCES

1. Duarte CS, Bordin IA, Yazigi L, et al. Factors associated with stress in mothers of children with autism. Autism 2005;9:416–27.
2. Montes G, Halterman JS. Characteristics of school-age children with autism. J Dev Behav Pediatr 2006;27:379–85.
3. Hastings RP, Kovshoff H, Ward NJ, et al. Systems analysis of stress and positive perceptions in mothers and fathers of pre-school children with autism. J Autism Dev Disord 2005;35:635–44.
4. Hastings RP, Daley D, Burns C, et al. Maternal distress and expressed emotion: cross sectional and longitudinal relationships with behavior problems of children with intellectual disabilities. Am J Ment Retard 2006;111:48–61.
5. Lounds J, Seltzer MM, Greenberg JS, et al. Transition and change in adolescents and young adults with autism: longitudinal effects on maternal well-being. Am J Ment Retard 2007;112:401–17.
6. Smith M, Philippen LR. Community integration and supported employment. In: Zager D, editor. Autism spectrum disorders: identification, education, and treatment. 3rd edition. Mahwah (NJ): Lawrence; 2005. p. 493–514.
7. Seltzer MM, Shattuck P, Abbeduto L, et al. The trajectory of developments in adolescents and adults with autism. Ment Retard Dev Disabil Res Rev 2004; 34:41–8.

8. Shattuck PT, Seltzer MM, Greenberg JS, et al. Change in autism symptoms and maladaptive behaviors in adolescents and adults with an autism spectrum disorder. J Autism Dev Disord 2007;37:1735–47.

9. Smith LE, Hong J, Seltzer MM, et al. Daily experiences among mothers of adolescents and adults with ASD. J Autism Dev Disord 2010;40:167–78.

10. Smith LE, Seltzer MM, Greenberg JS. Daily health symptoms of mothers of adolescents and adults with fragile X syndrome and mothers of adolescents and adults with autism spectrum disorder. J Autism Dev Disord 2012;42: 1836–46.

11. Seltzer MM, Greenberg JS, Hong J, et al. Maternal cortisol levels and behavior problems in adolescents and adults with ASD. J Autism Dev Disord 2010;40: 457–69.

12. Butzlaff RL, Hooley JM. Expressed emotion and psychiatric relapse: a meta analysis. Arch Gen Psychiatry 1998;55:547–52.

13. Leff JP, Vaughn CE. Expressed emotion in families. New York: Guilford Press; 1985.

14. Brown GW, Birley JL, Wing JK. Influence of family life on the course of schizophrenic disorders: a replication. Br J Psychiatry 1972;121:241–58.

15. Hooley JM. Expressed emotion and relapse of psychopathology. Annu Rev Clin Psychol 2007;3:329–52.

16. Wearden AJ, Tarrier N, Barrowclough C, et al. A review of expressed emotion in health care. Clin Psychol Rev 2000;20:633–66.

17. Kwon J, Delaney-Black V, Covington C, et al. The relations between maternal expressed emotion and children's perceived self-competence, behavior and intelligence in African-American families. Early Child Dev Care 2006;176: 195–206.

18. Wedig MM, Nock MK. Parental expressed emotion and adolescent self-injury. J Am Acad Child Adolesc Psychiatry 2007;46:1171–8.

19. Beck A, Daley D, Hastings RP, et al. Mother's expressed emotion towards children with and without intellectual disabilities. J Intellect Disabil Res 2004; 48:628–38.

20. Chadwick OO, Kusel YY, Cuddy MM. Factors associated with the risk of behaviour problems in adolescents with severe intellectual disabilities. J Intellect Disabil Res 2008;52:864–76.

21. Peris T, Baker B. Applications of the expressed emotion construct to young children with externalizing behavior: stability and prediction over time. J Child Psychol Psychiatry 2000;41:457–62.

22. Peris TS, Hinshaw SP. Family dynamics and preadolescent girls with ADHD: the relationship between expressed emotion, ADHD symptomatology, and comorbid disruptive behavior. J Child Psychol Psychiatry 2003;44:1177–90.

23. Baker BL, Heller TL, Henker B. Expressed Emotion, parenting stress, and adjustment in mothers of young children with behavior problems. J Child Psychol Psychiatry 2000;41:907–15.

24. Hastings RP, Lloyd T. Expressed emotion in families of children and adults with intellectual disabilities. Ment Retard Dev Disabil Res Rev 2007;13:339–45.

25. Barker ET, Hartley SL, Seltzer MM, et al. Trajectories of emotional well-being in mothers of adolescents and adults with autism. Dev Psychol 2011;47: 551–61.

26. Seltzer MM, Greenberg JS, Taylor JL, et al. Adolescents and adults with autism spectrum disorder. In: Amaral DG, Dawson G, Geschwind D, editors. Autism spectrum disorders. New York: Oxford University Press; 2011. p. 241–52.

27. Lord C, Rutter M, Le Couteur A. Autism Diagnostic Interview-Revised: a revised version of a diagnostic interview for caregivers of individuals with possible pervasive developmental disorders. J Autism Dev Disord 1994;24:659–85.

28. Magaña AB, Goldstein MJ, Karno M, et al. A brief method for assessing expressed emotion in relatives of psychiatric patients. Psychiatry Res 1986; 17:203–12.

29. Bruininks RH, Woodcock RW, Weatherman RF, et al. Scales of independent behavior – revised. Itasca (IL): Riverside Publishing; 1996.

30. Greenberg JS, Seltzer MM, Hong J, et al. Bidirectional effects of expressed emotion and behavior problems and symptoms in adolescents and adults with autism. Am J Ment Retard 2006;111:229–49.

31. Baker JK, Smith LE, Greenberg JS, et al. Change in maternal criticism and behavior problems in adolescents and adults with autism across a 7-year period. J Abnorm Psychol 2011;120:465–75.

32. Greenberg J, Mailick MR, Smith LE, et al. Bidirectional effects of the family environment and behavior problems in children, adolescents, and adults with fragile X syndrome. under review.

33. Achenbach T, Rescorla LA. Manual for the ASEBA school-age forms & profile: an integrated system of multi-informant assessments. Burlington (VT): University of Vermont, Research Center for Children, Youth, Families; 2001.

34. Achenbach TM, Rescorla LA. Manual for ASEBA adult forms & profiles. Burlington (VT): University of Vermont, Research Center for Children, Youth, Families; 2003.

35. Smith LE, Greenberg JS, Seltzer MM, et al. Symptoms and behavior problems of adolescents and adults with autism: effects of mother-child relationship quality, warmth, and praise. Am J Ment Retard 2008;113:387–402.

36. Taylor J, Seltzer M. Changes in the autism behavioral phenotype during the transition to adulthood. J Autism Dev Disord 2010;40:1431–46.

37. Taylor J, Seltzer M. Changes in the mother-child relationship during the transition to adulthood for youth with autism spectrum disorder. J Autism Dev Disord 2011; 41:1397–410.

38. Cox MJ, Paley B. Families as systems. Annu Rev Psychol 1997;48:243–67.

39. Hogarty GE, Anderson CM, Reiss DJ, et al. Family psychoeducation, social skills training, and maintenance chemotherapy in the aftercare treatment of schizophrenia: II. Two-year effects of a controlled study on relapse and adjustment. Arch Gen Psychiatry 1991;48:340–7.

40. Klaus N, Fristad MA. Family psychoeducation as a valuable adjunctive intervention for children with bipolar disorder. Dir Psychiatr 2005;25:217–30.

41. Lukens EP, McFarlane WR. Psychoeducation as evidence-based practice: considerations for practice, research, and policy. In: Roberts AR, Yeager KR, editors. Foundations of evidence-based social work practice. Oxford (United Kingdom): Oxford University Press; 2006. p. 291–313.

42. McFarlane WR, Hornby H, Dixon L, et al. Psychoeducational multifamily groups: research and implementation in the United States. In: Lefley HP, Johnson DL, editors. Family interventions in mental illness: international perspectives. Westport (CT): Praeger Publishers/Greenwood Publishing Group; 2002. p. 43–60.

43. Dixon L, Adams C, Lucksted A. Update on family psychoeducation for schizophrenia. Schizophr Bull 2000;26:5–20.

44. McFarlane WR, Dixon L, Lukens E, et al. Family psychoeducation and schizophrenia: a review of the literature. J Marital Fam Ther 2003;29:223–45.

45. Colom F, Vieta E, Martinez-Aran A, et al. A randomized trial on the efficacy of group psychoeducation in the prophylaxis of recurrences in bipolar patients whose disease is in remission. Arch Gen Psychiatry 2003;60:402–7.

46. Miklowitz DJ, George EL, Richards JA, et al. A randomized study of family-focused psychoeducation and pharmacotherapy in the outpatient management of bipolar disorder. Arch Gen Psychiatry 2003;60:904–12.

47. Rea MM, Tompson MC, Milowitz DJ, et al. Family-focused treatment versus individual treatment for bipolar disorder: results of a randomized clinical trial. J Consult Clin Psychol 2003;71:482–92.

48. Smith LE, Greenberg JS, Mailick MR. Adults with autism: outcomes, family effects, and multi-family group psychoeducaiton model. Curr Psychiatry Rep 2012;14:732–8.

49. Cohen S, Williamson G. Perceived stress in a probability sample of the United States. In: Spacapan S, Oskamp S, editors. The social psychology of health: Claremont symposium on applied social psychology. Newbury Park (CA): Sage; 1988. p. 31–67.

50. Constantino JN, Davis SA, Todd RD, et al. Validation of a brief quantitative measure of autistic traits: comparison of the social responsiveness scale with autism diagnostic interview-revised. J Autism Dev Disord 2003;33:I427–33.

51. Smith L, Maenner M, Seltzer M. Developmental trajectories in adolescents and adults with autism: the case of daily living skills. J Am Acad Child Adolesc Psychiatry 2012;51(6):622–31.

52. Smith LE, Mailick MR, Greenberg JS. Interpersonal relationships and social participation as markers of quality of life of adolescents and adults with autism and fragile X syndrome. under review.

53. Taylor JL, Mailick MR. A Longitudinal Examination of 10-Year Change in Vocational and Educational Activities for Adults With Autism Spectrum Disorders. Developmental Psychology 2013. http://dx.doi.org/10.1037/a0034297. Advance online publication.

54. Esbensen AJ, Bishop S, Seltzer M, et al. Comparisons between individuals with autism spectrum disorders and individuals with down syndrome in adulthood. Am J Intellect Dev Disabil 2010;115:277–90.

55. Cappadocia MC, Weiss JA, Pepler D. Bullying experiences among children and youth with autism spectrum disorders. J Autism Dev Disord 2012;42:266–77.

56. Montes G, Halterman JS. Bullying among children with autism and the influence of comorbidity with ADHD: a population-based study. Ambul Pediatr 2007;7: 253–7.

57. Van Roekel E, Scholte R, Didden R. Bullying among adolescents with autism spectrum disorders: prevalence and perception. J Autism Dev Disord 2010; 40:63–73.

Index

Note: Page numbers of article titles are in **boldface** type.

Child Adolesc Psychiatric Clin N Am 23 (2014) 157–165
http://dx.doi.org/10.1016/S1056-4993(13)00099-0
1056-4993/14/$ – see front matter © 2014 Elsevier Inc. All rights reserved.
childpsych.theclinics.com

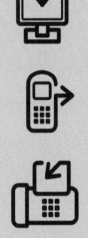